Narrative Meditation

Narrative Meditation

Remembering the Self

Terry Clancy

To order additional copies of this book, contact:
Xlibris
1-800-455-039
www.Xlibris.com.au
Orders@Xlibris.com.au
786328

Contents

This book is dedicated to those who inspired this story
My parents, daughters, friends, teachers
And Binda my constant companion.

Introduction

There are different ways to practice meditation. This book is about the method of Narrative Meditation. Meditation is a neuroplastic exercise of change in awareness and experience through self healing. It is learnt in three stages.

The meditation is on constructing a pyramid through change in awareness. The stages of constructing it are deeper levels of meditation. The deeper levels are different levels of experience as healing. Self healing can be understood as curing a problem. In a strength based approach, self healing means maximising our potential. Meditation is accessed through self healing of the levels to maximise our potential for health, well being and happiness.

Science is saying we, the universe, our environment are energy fields. It has to be otherwise we would not exist. Our bodies, emotions, thoughts and beliefs, and our environment are energy; we are energy fields. This is the most profound thought to the curious. This remains just a thought unless awareness that we are energy fields has purpose for our experience. We can either let science work out the implications of that or it can lead us to an interesting question; how can we intentionally maximise our potential through using our energy field? What is our energy field, and how do we access and use it are the questions.

The state of meditation is not defined. It is thought of as being a religious or mystical experience or as a state of quantum consciousness which mean different things to different people. It needs to be defined to access it and it's benefits. The state of meditation is accessed through the transformative vision. It is through understanding this transformative vision as having meaning and purpose that we access its benefits for health and well being. The connection of meditation, self healing, and experience with beliefs about that is transformative of our identity of who we are as individuals.

The meditation is on a pyramid. The pyramid is an integrated whole of it's framework of values as foundations, the seven inner levels of awareness, the four aspects of experience, and the apex where they all meet. The method is constructing it in stages as meditation deepens. Meditation deepens as understanding changes. Change in understanding is a change in awareness. The pyramid forms awareness of self. The levels of meditation as different levels of awareness are different levels of consciousness. This change in awareness changes our experience using meditation as a method of change and transformation.

This book was initiated by a friend. After reading my book, **As We Remember, Narrative Meditation and Vision,** he asked how do we use vision in everyday life? I had finished writing the book on my birthday. It was my gift to myself as a writer but I had not emphasised how vision is creating our experience in everyday life. Doing that now was significant to me as a guide, a writer and as a person. They were being connected as I was changing my lifestyle of how to be.

There are different layers of understanding the question. Vision is associated with prediction or prophecy. Prediction is awareness of current trends and predicting them converging in the future. Prophecy is predictions that are collectively agreed upon as the basis of religious faith. A book about remembering the self doesn't seem to fit as an answer but meditation, the self and experience are connected.

There are different opinions as to why this may occur as there are different paths of understanding the human psyche through reasoning of science, creativity of the arts, belief based on faith or transformation based on meditation. Narrative Meditation is a method learnt through self healing. Through self healing we remember what has been causing change is vision. Vision isn't about seeing with the senses, it's about knowingness; a change in consciousness. The self is state of consciousness of vision that changes our experience. The original question is the same as the question of what the self is.

I had my first experience of meditation through a guru 50 years ago but did not understand it to enable me to remember that experience again. He explained it from his own level of awareness, how he learnt it, his experience, culture of customs and beliefs and his objectives for self and others. Teachers, guides and books describe meditation from different perspectives as a method, a process, an outcome, and objectives. Meditation is described from these perspectives which make understanding difficult. I did not start practicing meditation for two decades. Narrative Meditation is accessible because there are different levels of it.

I was a mental health nurse and clinical manager of rehabilitation services for people with mental health disabilities; a very small and disadvantaged group. Nursing as the therapeutic use of self was practiced around the world for many decades. As practice was developing as a mental health nurse, I started meditation practice. Mental health nursing and meditation converged to assist change. Narrative Meditation is based on a mental health nursing practice of the therapeutic use of self. As mental health nurse the self is awareness of body and emotions, thoughts, and beliefs. Awareness of what the self is changed through this method of learning meditation. Narrative Meditation is a method, a process and an outcome connected with objectives of healing.

My path of understanding the self took a long time. The first objective of this book is that understanding won't take a long time for you. The self is the energy of vision accessed through meditation and used as mindfulness of goals. The second objective of this book is accessing the state of meditation. The state of meditation is accessed through the transformative vision. Understanding the self is a change in awareness that gives the transformative vision meaning and purpose. Through having meaning and purpose we access meditation and healing.

The self is very close to us, only forgotten. As we remember the self we are using our energy field in daily living. Using this energy in daily living maximises our potential. This is possible because meditation and mindfulness are learnt in stages of remembering the opening of the levels. Remembering is a neuroplastic exercise of change in awareness that changes our experience. Secondly it can be learnt because we have strengths of creativity and reasoning and objectives of physical and mental well being. Thirdly Narrative Meditation is accessible because there are different levels of it. The different levels of healing are different levels of awareness of self.

Stories have meaning and purpose as they are connected as a whole. Our lives as a story is the same. It's how we understand it that makes the all the difference between it being memories or a narrative that is unfolding. The narrative unfolds as our stories of awareness, experience, and belief are connected as psyches transformation. Psyche is only transformed through stories. The self is remembered as our stories are connected.

This book started out as the final chapter and conclusion that should have been. It ended up as a book that connected the three. My first book was about how the experience of learning meditation changes awareness. The second was about how awareness of the transformative vision changes experience. This book as the final chapter of a narrative that had been unfolding is a story of the remembering of the self.

Awareness

The story begins with awareness. Neuroscience is saying that consciousness changes because the brain is plastic; it changes structure and functioning as awareness changes. Our experience of self and environment, our reality is a construct of change in awareness.

Awareness, consciousness, and mind are terms used interchangeably with psyche. Awareness is consciousness; consciousness is mind. They are interacting with psyche but are not the same thing. Psyche is awareness of body and mind of emotions, thoughts and beliefs that form our identity. Awareness changes as we reflect on experience. Mind is a mirror of our awareness of self and environment. That's the development of who we are as people and what psyche is; our identity.

I was a mental health nurse and clinical manager for 38 years. Roles changed as awareness changed as I asked myself why does change occur, what is doing it better, how to do it better and what is the self? As a beginning practitioner mental health nurse, experience was changing awareness of self. As a nurse the self is awareness of body, thoughts, emotions and beliefs. Awareness changes when there is purpose. As a nurse the purpose is the therapeutic use of self in service of others. In meditation the purpose is the opening of the levels.

As a student I learnt the challenging nursing theory of Martha Rogers in the 70's that self and environment are interconnected energy fields. It challenged my understanding of who I was as an individual. In her theory movement into the unified environmental energy field occurs through self healing. We self heal through meditation but why self healing happens needed to be understood, how to do that had to be put into practice and what was the outcome of identity as unitary man?

I knew through experience that body and mind of thoughts, emotions and beliefs are interacting and a holistic model had real outcomes of health but they needed to be put into practice through developing a method of change. My roles as a nurse changed as clinical skills improved, were integrated with awareness of self and were put into practice. They were put into practice through participating in developing a model of care and service planning that I was involved with for two decades.

The improvement mirrored change in outer circumstances of policy and community expectations, inner circumstances of experience with different methods, service need to improve, and awareness of how change occurs.

Recovery from mental illness is a process, an outcome, and objectives using a method of care planning. As a method, based on patient goals and objectives it changed my nursing practice. As an intervention it was meaningful, provided continuity of care and could be taught to new staff. Nursing practice is also about teaching methods of healing to others.

The care plan was a holistic assessment of the key principles of recovery, planning through goals to achieve objectives, and implementation and review in partnership with the patient; that's the nursing process. With the seriously mentally ill, the problem isn't just the treatment resistant illness; it is compounded by physical, emotional, social, and cognitive problems that are interacting and need to be assessed. Through the method of care planning of assessment using principles, and implementation through goals to achieve objectives, recovery is achieving a meaningful life. Symptom management strategies and risks were included in the plan that was reviewed to keep them in mind. What is recovered is identity.

Nurses would ask how to do a care plan. I would ask them what is currently happening? One nurse said her patient had activities of daily living, symptom management strategies that he used when he was feeling stressed, was seeing his doctors regularly, was walking and talking with him daily and reviewing the plan with him weekly. What was changing was lifestyle and well being. What is forming through the plan is vision of a meaningful life. This vision forms through awareness of change occurring. I said if he agrees with his plan, document it and get it approved by the team. It was about a plan that had meaning not using psychiatric jargon which patients don't understand.

One day that very gentle man gave me a rugby style tackle which was amusing for those who were watching. His medications had been changed and hyperactivity was a side effect. An expert nurse is always assessing even at ground level. The care plan changed as circumstances changed to keep them dynamic sources of healing. I went to hear her care plan presentation. Successful care planning is about empowerment of others.

The plan was about hope for present and future well being that was shared between patient and nurse; the basis of the therapeutic alliance was vision of a meaningful life. The work of a mental health nurse was the therapeutic use of self to assist others to achieve this vision. We use self through becoming self aware. We assist others using the method of care planning as a model of change.

The forming of goals involves using reasoning and creativity to remember them as experience. All rehabilitation programs involve goals for the present and objectives for the future. I was becoming a better nurse through assisting mindfulness of goals and objectives as a process of change in awareness and experience.

Patients who either had long term serious mental illnesses, challenging behaviours and intellectual handicap or were a possible threat to themselves or others had improved outcomes of decrease in symptoms, and life skills to achieve the objective of community integration.

As a strength based approach the care plan is not a focus on problems. Recovery from mental illness occurred through using strengths. The method of care planning developed mindfulness of goals and what was previously stressful was coped with. As recovery occurred mental health crises were prevented. The point is the method of change in working for the seriously mentally ill, can work for most people.

The therapeutic use of self was learnt through reflective practice, clinical supervision, performance appraisal, career pathways, interaction with patients and working with psychiatrists as team leaders for over twenty years. Knowingness of when and how to assist others is the art of mental health nursing that can't be taught; it is only learnt through experience. Care planning is the evidence base of practice of a recovery focussed nurse.

I became aware of neuroplasticity in the 80s when I cared for an adolescent with acquired brain injury. Half of his brain had been severely damaged, a consequence of a cerebral haematoma at birth. He had successfully completed high school but had developed emotional outbursts. After assessment the psychiatrist informed the family the functioning half had taken over the other half's functions. The problem was he was an adolescent who needed limits set on his behaviour, not medicating. His brain had changed structure and functioning throughout his life in response to learning. The plan was for him to become aware of and responsible for his behaviour within a supportive environment. The therapeutic objective is recovery of a meaningful life secure in his identity as an adolescent. His behaviour changed after 2 months and so did that of most others.

Care planning as a formal structured approach to rehabilitation is a neuroplastic intervention of change in awareness and experience based on care planning as model of change. The vision of a meaningful life is the recovery of identity; that's what recovery means. People engaged in rehabilitation goals, objectives and with others when this was understood.

I was a clinical manager for 23 years which was about the development of new services. My role as manager was organising services based on vision of collective well being of target patient populations. That was achieved using principles of recovery orientated services formalised as a plan. The parts of the services were connected as a whole through operational planning.

There is a difference between planning and management of crisis. The difference is preventing crises occurring through root cause analysis of trends and the old methods of reacting were no longer working in an environment that was rapidly changing. Through goals and objectives better service outcomes were achieved and individual crises prevented. Operational planning as best practice management worked too; that's what governance is all about.

As I was becoming a nursing consultant and manager, I was learning change management at university. Through experiential learning I learnt a model of change through goals and objectives to achieve the vision of what the organisation was about. Goals and objectives of the parts linked the organisation as a whole. Vision makes a difference to organisation, to individuals, groups and communities. Nursing and management were interrelated as the development of models of change using principles, goals, and objectives to achieve a vision.

The first axiom of being a healer in any capacity is to self heal. As my clinical skills improved, I was developing a meditation method. Developing a method was about developing a model that had meaning and purpose in my circumstances, and level of knowledge and skills in meditation.

Assessment, planning through goals, and implementation and review in partnership with the patient is the nursing process. The meditation is self assessment, planning through goals and implementation and review of opening of the levels as a method of change. The levels have meaning as principles and purpose as goals that can be imagined as experience. Meditation practice is remembering the plan to either solidify or change goals as needed. I was developing a method to self heal and in doing so change experience for self and others if needed.

My model of mental health nursing practice was the basis of developing my meditation. Meditation on the levels develops awareness of self. Mental health nursing is the use of self. They converged as awareness of and using self to heal. The method of care planning was a model of change to assist others heal. In Roger's theory we move into the unified environmental energy field through self healing. We self heal through meditation. Narrative Meditation as a model of change is a method of self healing. Self healing occurs through using our strengths of reasoning and creativity to be who we want to be. Awareness of what the self is at the 8th level is a change in awareness of who we are.

Awareness of self was changing through the method of meditation. Empowerment can move immoveable mountains of doubt and regret. We are empowered through change occurring. Empowerment through change occurring is well being. As a method it is a neuroplastic exercise of change in awareness of self.

∞

Narrative meditation is a method of using the pyramid as a symbol to imagine our whole selves as levels of awareness. The pyramid has foundations of primary values of peace, love and beauty, four aspects of body, emotions, thoughts and beliefs, an unconscious inside of levels of awareness that form them and an apex where they, what we are aware of and what we were not, meet as our whole selves.

Through the method awareness is changing. The apex of awareness is the transformative vision. The pyramid is symbolic of what is timeless and enduring, our unconscious image of unity with environment and wholeness of self. The apex is symbolic of intuitive awareness of ourself as whole.

Experience and awareness are relative, one is changing the other. Through the experience of opening of the levels we become self aware. Awareness develops from awareness of environment to awareness of self through reflection and meditation on goals of inner experience of opening of the levels. Goals are for the present moment; objectives are achieved through goals. Self awareness is mindfulness of goals and objectives in the present moment. To be mindful of goals is to remember them using this method of meditation.

∞

The levels of the pyramid open as they have meaning and purpose. They have meaning as principles based on values. The eight principles are; body and service, emotions and compassion, thoughts and creativity, belief and inner peace, love and presence, connection and beauty, spirit and others, union and identity. The principles of the levels developed through them having meaning as a holistic model and purpose of how to live. Meditation and lifestyle are connected. What connects them are goals.

Principles have purpose as goals of the levels. Goals develop using reasoning to mediate between them and creativity to imagine them as experience. The levels are opened, are accessed through imagining goals of healing of the levels as experience. Imagining something as experience is different from visualising something. Imagining is seeing through the mind's eye, feeling, believing, knowing the experience as happening. Through using mind the inner experience is remembered.

The levels of awareness as principles and goals are different state of consciousness that are transforming the outer aspects. The levels, principles, goals and the aspects of self are interrelated and dynamic; are changing. The principles changed in meaning as goals of healing developed as priorities for health and well being. That's how the method developed as the visualisation of the levels as colours, contemplation of their meaning as principles, and imagining goals of healing of the levels as experience. The meditation is on goals of our whole selves. The method of imagining goals of healing as experience is an internal technology of change and a neuroplastic exercise of change in awareness.

∞

Narrative Meditation is learnt in three stages of building upon the method before. Each stage is a meditation on the energy field as both individual, between us and the universal, unified energy field. The three stages are the forming of goals. There are three pyramids of four, seven and eight levels; the upper of each being a deeper level of meditation. At the first two levels we are the observer of change as the levels open and build upon each other. The third level of meditation is an integration of the methods where we are not the observer. A different narrative has been evolving through our stories.

Where do the colours of the levels come in? I did meditation on the levels as colours, sounds and mantras. I could not relate however to the chakras as physical energy centres within the body. I believe they are the energy of connection of neuronal brain maps. They reconnect as we remember the experience. In different meditation methods colours are associated with different levels of consciousness as energies. I did not know what the higher levels meant as more than colours. I meditated on them as colours till I did. They were accessed as they had meaning as principles and purpose as goals that could be imagined as experience; that's the method.

Colours are brain neurostimulators. Brain maps are neuronal connections being made that sweep like waves of energy across the brain. In this method the colours are linked with principles, goals, and objectives of healing of the levels. I think of it as the colour coding of awareness. In meditation the colours are associated with goals in the present moment. The colours like goals build upon one another and merge at the apex as the colour white.

Mindfulness is remembering goals. I use mindfulness of the colour green to relax my body, calm emotions, and still thoughts when in the dentist's chair. I don't like invasive procedures. I was interested in practical applications of meditation in everyday life. Different levels of meditation can be accessed in different circumstances. In awareness of the first level we are aware of and interact with our environment. At deeper levels we don't. By remembering the colours we create the inner experience in the present moment.

In science, different cultures and in myth light has different meanings. The light of the shining star we associate with the universe. In physics light are particle waves of energy that the senses and brain perceives as light. Colloquially we speak of seeing the light as a euphemism for understanding. Enlightenment is the resolution of the problem of what seem opposites. The problem of everyday life and the problem of understanding self are resolved as we self heal. Attaining a certain lightness of being is the objective of self healing. That's what the transformative vision does and is and what I think enlightenment means; awareness of our wholeness and unity, the transformative vision of the primary archetypal image.

As a meditation, the pyramid is symbolic of our whole selves. It is constructed using creativity of the imagination and reasoning. The meditation is on our whole selves as levels of awareness. The apex of awareness is the goal of inner experience of the transformative vision of the energy field; a higher level of awareness of connection.

Neuroplasticity is defined as the brain changing structure and functioning in response to activity and experience. (Doidge; **The Brain that Changes Itself.** p xv). Learning meditation is mental practice of using reasoning and the creativity of the imagination. Doidge describes using the imagination as a neuroplastic exercise. Imagining and experiencing with the senses have the same effects on the brain. (p214)

Artists and athletes in many fields use the imagination to improve mental and physical performance. Australian Stephanie Gilmore used visualisation to imagine herself winning the Bells Beach championship; she did and has won the World Surfing Championship six times. All successful people use the imagination. What distinguishes them is mindfulness of goals and objectives. Ask any coach if awareness of goals, objectives and possibilities (being in a representative team is a possibility) are important for success in their respective fields. Awareness that our field is energy is important for success in creating health and well being.

The opening of the levels is changing awareness. The method of meditation is a neuroplastic exercise of change in awareness through imagining goals of healing of the levels as experience. We know the method and why change to the aspects is occurring but what is doing that?

∞

Archaeologists attempt to understand the pyramids of Giza as structures that had meaning and purpose in antiquity. That becomes know as they question why they were important, how they were built and what they symbolised. The pyramids of Giza were built in layers one upon the other forming the outer aspects. The meditation is on the pyramid being constructed through change in awareness that open the inner levels. Meditation is a level of awareness that deepens in stages. Remembering the experience of their opening is building upon the others. Building upon the others is through change in awareness

Meditation is usually described as a process, 'I went into meditation on...', but what is the process? Memories are the recollection of experiences encoded in the brain. The most effective way to remember is practicing the experience in the mind. I wanted to remember the experience of meditation again by trying different meditation methods. We remember the experience using reasoning and creativity. That's the process of change in awareness. Creativity is imagining it; inspiration is opening of the levels through goals; knowingness is awareness of it occurring.

Consciousness develops as awareness of self and environment changes. Full consciousness is the integration of what we are aware of, and what we were not. What we are not consciously aware of is that we are energy fields. Principles and goals of the levels are different states of consciousness of awareness of self and environment as energy fields. As what was unconscious becomes known, mind is being transformed. Mind is transformed as the unconscious archetypal image becomes known and we know how to access it and use it.

The opening of the levels is occurring using reasoning and creativity of the imagination. Full consciousness develops through awareness of goals of the levels. The unified energy field isn't seen with the senses, it is known imagining the transformative vision. The transformative vision is intuitive awareness of the energy field. This change in awareness is through the development of creativity as imagination, inspiration and intuition. Full consciousness is the integration of reasoning that we are energy fields with intuitive awareness of it. The mind's eye, its way of knowing is intuition. The levels of awareness are different states of consciousness building upon each other. Awareness changes as we meditate on goals of the levels. The goal of inner experience of the transformative vision is a change in consciousness as intuition. Intuition is a state of knowingness of connections existing.

People experience intuition as synchronistic experiences that mirror consciousness and serendipity, outer circumstances falling into place. They demonstrate to us there is more to our experience than just our thoughts. On the separate paths of understanding through reasoning, creativity, and faith, people experience intuition as inspiration, as peaks of connection of consciousness and experience.

Inspiration is the energy of connection of new brain maps occurring. I notice that when inspired by goals my energy level increased and inner and outer circumstances fell into place; I was in the flow of experience. On the path of meditation, reasoning has changed and creativity has developed as intuition. It wasn't spontaneous for me unfortunately, but homeostasis occurs as we are made whole. I had an inspiration it could be spontaneous for others through understanding the transformative vision, but that's an objective we are yet to arrive at.

Carl Jung believed that intuition was the cause of external synchronistic experiences and serendipitous events and that the cause had to be energy but could not link intuition with energy. Joseph Campbell, an expert on mythology had a feeling that mind and energy are the same thing; that our life force is the energy of consciousness that is transformed by the understanding of myths and meditation. (**The Power of Myth**, p.14) Both could not say what the energy source was or how it is used to maximises our potential. What is the connection of synchronistic appearance of a Scarab beetle on a window, Psyche's story of transformation through achieving her goals, the archetypal images, and our own health and well being? The connection is energy. Energy is any force that produces change to inner and outer circumstances. Consciousness is energy when it produces change. To be energy it has to be intentionally used to heal.

The energy field is known through the development of reasoning and intuition as full consciousness. We can access this energy as an intention. Full consciousness is more than knowingness. Full consciousness is intentionally accessing this energy through mindfulness of goals. Meditation is a method of developing awareness of our whole selves as goals and a process of the transformation of mind as full consciousness. Full consciousness is mindfulness of goals of our whole selves. Consciousness changes as we remember the experience of meditation; that's where neuroplasticity comes in and why regular practice is necessary for change to occur.

On the inner journey the opening of the levels is changing awareness. The ending of the inner journey is awareness of the transformative vision. This change in awareness is a change in consciousness. The different levels of meditation are different levels of awareness of self and environment as energy fields. Meditation deepens as the energy field becomes known. The process is the development of strengths of reasoning as beliefs, skills in meditation, knowledge of self and environment changes, and creativity evolves using the imagination. Change occurs through using our strengths. The method is meditation on the pyramid but the process is a change in awareness as full consciousness as what was unconscious becomes known. Awareness changes through remembering the experience of opening of the levels and we use it as mindfulness of goals of the levels.

∞

Science is saying that the universe is an interconnected whole of energy but they don't say we as energy fields are part of it; that's what a cosmologist really is. I had read the spiritual theory that the universe was an energy field and that union with it occurs in the state of meditation. Deepak Chopra described how this state of consciousness causes healing at a quantum level of energy. I had learnt the nursing theory that through self healing we are made whole through awareness of the universal environmental energy field. Both linked meditation with healing.

Meditation is a method, and a process but what is it as an outcome? Meditation is usually understood as absence of awareness of body, emotions, thoughts and beliefs but it isn't. The different levels of meditation are accessed as goals of inner experience. The inner experience is remembered when it has meaning as goals and purpose as healing. Meditation deepens as the energy field becomes known. The different levels of meditation as different states of consciousness are different levels of healing.

The state of meditation is accessed as a goal of inner experience of the transformative vision. The transformative vision as intuition is an outcome of the method and the process of transformation of consciousness. I had experienced meditation and wanted to remember it again. I had the experience again as I understood what it was as a different state of consciousness and how I could access it. Another level of awareness is opened as we do. That's the process of opening of the levels.

We are part of a unified energy field that has always existed, and through its transformation always will. The unified field is an interconnected whole of energy across time and space. The unified field transforms only. In this method awareness of the unified field is through the transformative vision. In meditation the colours of the levels merge as a wave of light. This light is not experienced by the senses, it is known in the imagination. The transformative vision is light that transcends the past, present and future. The exercise is brain being aware of the experience of union with the energy field.

Awareness of the unified field is through the transformative vision of the past, present and future meeting. Where they meet there is no time or space as distance between objects. There are no objects because objects are located in time. Space and time are transcended by the goal of inner experience of the transformative vision. The transformative vision is the state of meditation where there is no time or objects. The state of meditation is the transformative vision of the unified field. Where there are objects there is time. That is how you end the meditation on the transformative vision, by awareness of time and space as objects.

∞

Narrative meditation is a method of change, a process of transformation of consciousness, an outcome of the transformative vision, and objectives we have of it. I talk to people who say they never got anything out of meditation; to clarify that, I ask what did they want to achieve? There are different reasons as to why we practice meditation, different objectives. The method, the process and outcomes are connected with objectives we have of it. Objectives give meditation purpose. There are different objectives of the levels of meditation. Leant in stages makes meditation accessible but objectives change as understanding changes and we ask more questions.

Most people want only to listen to a guided meditation to relax. It is not about understanding it as a method, reaching higher levels of awareness or change. I did guided meditations for others as a stress management strategy. It was not about accessing deeper levels of meditation. Deeper levels require involvement in it as a neuroplastic exercise of change. The guided meditations were effective but not for change in awareness, experience, beliefs or longer term lifestyle change. Mindfulness may be your objective but then we get curious and start asking questions. Narrative Meditation is a method of change and transformation through self healing as an objective.

Talking to a person about meditation, I explained it firstly as learning breath control to relax the body, calm the emotions and still the thoughts and that the meditation is on this state of inner peace; the first meditation. He said meditation is just about relaxation; I said yes it is about the goal of relaxation but also about mindfulness of relaxation as an objective in everyday life. Guided meditations, breath control and relaxation may be your objective. By practicing them we are using mindfulness of goals.

Meditation is accessible because there are different levels of it. The different levels have different objectives. The three stages of learning meditation have different objectives of individual, transpersonal and spiritual healing. Objectives change as the higher levels are opened through them having meaning as principles and purpose as goals. Meditation deepens as the energy field becomes known. It becomes known as understanding changes. Change in understanding is a change in awareness.

The first meditation is on the peace of inner silence as the first three levels are healed through goals of relaxation, calm, and stillness of thought; meditation on the peace of inner silence at the fourth level is an objective of individual healing.

The second meditation on the seventh level is accessed through goals of unconditional love, connection with environment, and awareness of the energy field as love between us. In meditation on this goal of connection the objective is healing at a transpersonal level. The third meditation is the goal of inner experience of the transformative vision; intuitive awareness of union with the universal energy field is an objective of spiritual healing; awareness of our wholeness and unity. Beliefs and objectives are changing as we self heal.

We recover from loss through inspirational goals in the present for the future. It's what we do throughout life to heal. Remembering goals for the present and future is also a forgetting. We don't deny the loss, it happened, we are replacing the experiences associated with it using our strengths to imagine goals for the present and future. It's how ordinary people in everyday life get over loss and trauma; but they aren't ordinary; they also have beliefs about that.

We recover from loss of awareness of self through self healing of the levels. In a strength based approach, self healing means achieving goals of how we want to be; not a focus on problems. People used to say don't feed our problems energy. I believe that is literally true and how neuroplasticity can be made to work for us. The different levels of meditation have different objectives of self healing at an individual, transpersonal and spiritual level. The different levels are accessed as objectives and beliefs about self and environment changes.

The state of meditation is accessed through the transformative vision. Healing occurs through the experience. In meditation on the transformative vision of the unified field we are a mirror image of that of wholeness, of connection of our parts. This integration occurs through the transformation of consciousness at the apex of awareness. The pyramid is symbolic of our energy field as this whole self.

Through meditation consciousness is transformed as mindfulness of goals. Mindfulness of goals is an intention to heal. This gives the method of Narrative Meditation meaning as a neuroplastic exercise of change in awareness and purpose as self healing.

Mind is creative energy in awareness of the transformative vision of union with the energy field, and how we access this energy in mindfulness of goals in awareness of why; to realise the objectives of meditation practice. The objective of deeper levels of meditation is different levels of healing. Spiritual healing is awareness of the transformative vision of our wholeness and unity. Through self healing we are made whole but what are our parts and how are they connected?

∞

Awareness that we and environment are energy fields is the most profound thought. Before we accept that, it must be of use to us in daily living. After 4 billion years of evolution, what is the purpose of mind? Understanding has been the source of the evolution of mind and who we are as a species. The human brain miraculously evolved as we did. Consciousness developed through understanding our environment in order to survive through adaptation. The purpose is to maintain homeostasis, balance of the aspects of body, emotions, thoughts and beliefs to achieve and maintain health and well being. Doidge describes in his book **The Brain's Way of Healing** how through internal neuoroplastic neurostimulation, the brain is healed to modulate itself to achieve homeostasis.(p 109).

We are energy fields that balance the field to achieve homeostasis through self healing. Our whole self is an energy field that is the connection of our parts. Through the transformative vision of union with the energy field we are a mirror image of that of wholeness. The method is our internal technology of connecting our parts through self healing. Self healing through awareness of the levels is a change in consciousness. Consciousness is connecting our parts as an integrated whole in awareness of the transformative vision, the state of meditation.

∞

Do You Remember was about how the method of meditation on the levels of awareness developed. It concluded by remembering the transformative vision of wholeness and unity, a change in consciousness. **As We Remember** was about how through remembering the transformative vision experience changed in awareness of possibilities. The three possibilities of self healing are a renaissance of culture, the prevention of mental illness and vision. As we remember on the outer journey what has been transforming awareness, healing the levels, creating the experience of meditation, transforming the aspects of self, and opening up possibilities what is remembered is vision. Full consciousness as mindfulness of goals and objectives of our whole selves is vision. Psyche, identity is being transformed.

The turning point is using meditation as neuroplastic exercise to self heal. The omega point is a decision of how to be. Empowerment through change leads to engagement in meditation and mindfulness of goals. Where is this leading if mastery of Narrative Meditation is an objective and what is that?

Our stories are what we are learning from. Through them a different narrative is evolving. How we use vision in everyday life is through goals, objectives and possibilities that inspire. In our circumstances we have our roles but it is the art of how we carry them out that makes all the difference. In life synchronistic experiences and serendipitous events have purpose to assist fulfil our goals. The task is awareness of them, checking and balancing them using reasoning and that's what mind does. All experience becomes information needed to realise goals and objectives. The transformative vision of union is awareness that self and all things are connected.

The transformative vision is the state of meditation that makes whole. We are made whole through the connection of our framework of awareness, experience, and beliefs. Mastery of Narrative Meditation is a lifestyle decision of how to be made in awareness of how possibilities of vision are connecting our framework as an integrated whole.

Meditation is a personal art of change in lifestyle. There isn't meditation, goals, objectives and you. Meditation and lifestyle are integrated by goals to maximise our potential for well being. Mastery is more than being an expert, aware of the method, processes, outcomes and objectives. Mastery is a lifestyle decision of how to be. Vision is mindfulness of goals and objectives of our whole selves. Engagement in meditation and mindfulness leads to the transformation of consciousness as vision in everyday life; the fourth possibility.

Experience

I thought at times I had spiritually healed. A sage once said to followers that if you believe you are, you are not; which is true because the nature of the path of transformation is change in understanding. Understanding changes as meditation deepens. The opening of the levels were moments of inspiration, of breakthroughs that changed awareness, and experience.

I had experienced in meditation the opening of the 7th level. It occurred in a forest retreat I had built. It had a solid framework that consumed a lot of energy. As I was constructing it I experienced meditation as a state of awareness of connection of self with environment. For a decade I tried different methods to remember that experience again; I didn't. I had an experience of meditation but not the understanding of what it is, and how to remember it again. Remembering the experience is a change in awareness; and through that another level is opened. A different state of consciousness is accessed as we remember the experience.

I reflected on what the meditation was. I became aware that the apex is another level of awareness. That's what pyramids do; they change awareness. I did remember that experience again as an intention on a misty morning overlooking a valley from my window. Remembering is about recalling details. Meditation is a process of change in awareness that deepens as understanding changes.

The apex of awareness is a goal of inner experience of the transformative vision of union. The three levels of meditation as different levels of awareness of self and environment as energy fields are different intentions of healing. I had been waiting for the experience again. It happened again as a goal of inner experience of the transformative vision.

Pyramids are enigmatic. It is complex to understand why they were important, how they were constructed and what they symbolised; what was the intention? The meaning of the pyramids is understanding them as structures connected with their environment. As a meditation the meaning of the pyramid is changing and so is it's purpose as understanding of self and environment changes. Change in awareness changes our experience. As we are made whole we are creating a new experience as healing.

Mind is a mirror of awareness. Self awareness is a mirror through which we see ourselves. The mirror is clouded by identity as our roles obscuring what we are. Vision is a clear mirror and what is reflected is experience. The levels of meditation as levels of awareness are different states of consciousness and experience as healing. Remembering goals and objectives in meditation as mental practice is a neuroplastic exercise of change in awareness and experience. The method is an intention to develop awareness of and use our energy field to transform experience. As understanding changes awareness we are creating our experience as healing.

Doidge has described how neuroplasticity of the brain can be used to maximise our potential using different methods. According to Rogers we are made whole, healed as we move into the environmental energy field but why does meditation make us whole, how do we access it, and what is being whole? Unitary man is a change in awareness, but what is he/she as experience, what are beliefs about that and what does change in identity have to do with it? We are being made whole as we self heal through connection of our framework of awareness, experience, and belief. Healing occurs through their connection. Without understanding of why they are connected, what spiritual healing is, and how we achieve it unitary man is an ideal.

I became an expert nurse. I will be a better guide and writer as I connect meditation, the transformative vision and mindfulness of goals with change in experience. Change can either occur using a long way round or through using a method. Through using the method, transformation is possible as we connect our stories of awareness and experience and that is the evolving narrative of transformation of awareness of what we are and who we are as people.

∞

We are more than our parts and our roles in life so the question is, why do the aspects of self change? Meditation deepens as the energy field becomes known through awareness of connection with it. This change in awareness is a change in consciousness. Through self healing mind is transforming the aspects. Experience has four aspects of body, emotions, thoughts and beliefs. As a nurse the self was understood as awareness of them. Through meditation on principles, goals and objectives they are being transformed. They are being transformed by healing of the inner levels... Awareness and experience are transformed by vision. Narrative Meditation is a neuroplastic exercise with the objective of transformation of psyche as service, compassion, creativity, and belief that self and environment are interconnected energy fields.

The inner journey is to the transformative vision of the unified field. This change in awareness is the transformation of consciousness. The outer journey is change in objectives as experience changes. Reasoning has changed and creativity has developed as imagination, inspiration, intuition and vision. Vision developed through meditation and as mindfulness of goals in everyday life underlies all decisions, tasks and responsibilities as who we are. Who we are as experience is transformed as a mirror of vision; the fifth possibility of vision is the transformation of experience.

In meditation and mindfulness in everyday life we are using the creative energy of mind. Vision is creative energy, an intentional state of connection of self and self with environment. Inner experience of self healing and the transformation of the aspects of self are connected. Vision is a state of synchronicity of consciousness, inner experience of healing of the levels, and transformation of the outer aspects. Vision is changing experience through self healing of the levels as a neuroplastic exercise.

In meditation and mindfulness we are remembering goals of experience that are encoded in the brain. The brain in turn transforms the aspects of experience. It is all occurring because the brain changes structure and functioning as awareness changes as we remember the opening of the levels; that's what practice does.

Awareness is consciousness. Through self healing mind is transformed as full consciousness. Full consciousness as mindfulness of all goals of the levels in everyday life is vision of ourself as whole. Our whole self is a mirror of vision; what we are as energy is who we are as experience. The self is state of consciousness of vision of goals and objectives of the levels. What we are as an energy field is the self; the self is our energy field. Our energy field is consciousness. The pyramid is symbolic of the self as a state of quantum consciousness of vision. Psyche awareness of who we are is transformed.

∞

The unfolding of the self has been written about in myth as the hero's journey, in legends of King Arthur's vision of a new man as the basis of the culture of Camelot that heralds a new society and legends of the morning star's return. The morning star has never gone away. It's return is awareness that the morning star is as a symbol of the self's return that heralds a new day beginning.

Awareness of the connection of self and environment has been sung about. Music inspires feelings; words inspire thoughts; songs inspire feelings about thoughts once upon a time. Songs use images to express awareness of connection of consciousness and experience; the connection of self, self with others, and self with environment. The quest that is sung about is reaching that unreachable star no matter what it takes.

The journey is a voyage of consciousness on the sea of experience. That good ship can either be fun or rolling on a dark and lonely sea of breaking waves of experience. Are we helpless against the tide? On seeing a shooting star I thought of me like you trying to break into another world I never knew. Listen to the tide slowly turning washing all our heartache away. In moments, when time stood still, I was more than I thought I could be, in green waves or fields of gold, by still waters, when silence covered the sky, over a rainbow where dreams come true, on seeing the light in the sky as that bright star in heaven that lights our way home, and we imagine the world living as one, we open our minds for a different vision and nothing else matters, I was free. I have seen the light, I have changed my ways, (so it was said) but these are the days by the sparkling river or climbing a ladder to the stars into the light I know but cannot write and stairways can't be bought but with the sound of silence planted in my brain I think to myself what a wonderful world but then the singer asks in dismay why are 49 candles burning at Orlando?

Alienation can drive formation or anger in believing nobody else knows what it feels like to be on your own and with no direction as to how to get home the blame is projected on others. These events are collectively felt that change our awareness. The words and voices have gone into collective understanding these events as symptoms of a crisis caused by alienation; absence of belief that self and environment are connected; what inspirational artists believe and express.

∞

My friends are people who on their paths of reflection based on reasoning, creativity, faith and meditation inspired me. Where we connected was through inspiration in mindfulness of goals that were mutual. It's why we enjoy our friendship. What they inspired was remembering of the self. I was the self in awareness that they were the self. But it was not a decision for me of how to be as the self and experience were not yet connected.

The self is a bridge formed by the transformative vision of the past and future to change experience in the present. It is constructed to be of service to self and others. The transformative vision is awareness of our wholeness and unity as energy fields. As we remember the transformative vision in meditation our whole self is the connection of our parts. Awareness and experience are connected by the energy of vision of ourselves as whole. Reasoning is understanding why and how this occurs, but belief is necessary for it to happen.

BELIEFS

Meditation has been researched as to its benefits for health and well being but the results have not been conclusive. Many people have experienced different benefits of meditation but they can't be scientifically established. Complexity is caused by not understanding what the methods are, what are the effects on awareness and experience, what are beliefs about that, what did the person want to achieve, and what does identity have to do with it.

That vision is a state of quantum consciousness causing cellular change is not proven. Reviews by experts of current evidence suggest it may never be scientifically established that there is a state of quantum consciousness that can cause healing. (BBC Earth, February, 2017). Scientists have proved that the building blocks of the universe are quantum particles of energy. The interesting thing about the experiments on them was they could not be observed by scientists. (BBC Earth). The particle is energy that only exists through belief in it.

This raises several points. In my experience research also follows changes in practice outcomes. Florence Nightingale could not scientifically prove that cleanliness, fresh air, diet and light enhanced healing; it was a belief based on her own action research of her practice. The lamp of practice lights up research and always will. Research in deconstructing us as parts misses the integrated whole on which health depends and that depends on beliefs.

The question of whether vision is energy is whether neuroplastic changes to the brain are an outcome of quantum changes occurring at a cellular level. It may never be proven that vision is a state of quantum consciousness; it depends on our beliefs. I believe vision is energy because something exists because of its effects.

We are energy fields. Our life force is the energy of consciousness. To be energy it must produce change. Meditation is proven as a neuroplastic exercise that is changing brain structure and functioning. The source of this change has to be energy. The transformative vision in meditation and as a state of consciousness of vision is energy that changes consciousness and experience as healing. Neuroplastic changes to the brain are occurring as a mirror of the energy of vision. Neuroplastic changes are effects of vision as a state of quantum consciousness.

Energy has to be used and beliefs are necessary for it to be energy. All neuroplastic exercises are a change in awareness and experience through belief that they are connected. Belief focuses attention that is necessary for any type of neuroplastic healing. The neuroplastic exercise of transformation of awareness and experience is connected with beliefs about that. What are the possibilities of vision for the transformation of beliefs about self and the relationship of self to environment?

Change occurs because beliefs give meaning and purpose. Through giving meaning and purpose they 'capture' vision as energy. Neuroscience is saying that beliefs filter the brain's interpretation of information affecting both awareness and experience. Beliefs about self and the relationship of self to environment give meaning to experience and purpose to meditation as a method of change and transformation. Beliefs are necessary for all levels of healing.

∞

The opening of the first four levels is transforming the aspects of body as service, emotions as compassion, thoughts as creativity, and belief in our individual healing; the first level of meditation. The next three by belief in transpersonal healing occurring through presence, connection with environment, and connection with others; the second level of meditation. The transformative vision is belief in our spiritual healing. The aspect of belief is being transformed as the higher levels are opened through change in belief as individual, transpersonal, and spiritual healing.

Neuroscience says that beliefs are creating our experience; what we believe is what we get. As nurse the therapeutic alliance was connection with patients through goals, objectives and shared vision of a meaningful life. The extent of the alliance was mutual goal setting. Beliefs about that were not connected with religious beliefs. Beliefs about self and the relationship of self to others changes through experience. Therapists who were transformative had unique relationships with patients who otherwise had great difficulty forming relationships with others. They were still points of connection of the self and the self within others in an otherwise chaotic world. That world changed as the firm ground on which to stand changed.

I worked with different models as a manager; custodial, medical, rehabilitation, forensic, community and disability. My role was to understand how the models affected nursing practice which caused problems when any change was necessary. Nursing practice is regulated by professional standards, statutes and common law and I was responsible for interpreting and implementing them while organisational change was occurring.

I was yelled at by my superior nurse at a public forum for recommending care planning as a method of rehabilitation for people who had been institutionalised. The belief was that rehabilitation would occur by simply opening the doors like in an old movie. It wasn't resistance to change, it was facilitating change using a model based on best practice. There was no understanding of care planning as a method of rehabilitation; the vision of what the service was. I stuck to it by the way and was supported by all psychiatrists. It was an integration of the medical model of treatment and recovery through rehabilitation using strengths.

Where there is no vision to guide objectives, and goals or the art of change, the organisation is a matrix of conflict. That's not simply a reflection on the past the same is true of beliefs where there is no mutual understanding. We have models of ourselves and those are our beliefs.

All people have beliefs about self and the relationship of self to environment. Belief may be that we are genetically pre programmed at birth with different attitudes, creativity, and reasoning, believe that consciousness is the senses, that mind is for making decisions and experience is an outcome of cause and effect of reasoning, that we are a physical being living in a material universe governed by physics, motivated by self interest, and that consciousness ceases when the body dies.

In this system of beliefs, there is no connection of self and self with environment at higher levels of awareness and that is our self fulfilling reality of experience. They as a collective model are cultural beliefs. They are not religious beliefs but beliefs none the less that shapes our experience. Consciousness, experience and these beliefs are connected. What connects them is identity of psyche as ego formed through our culture.

Beliefs evolve; they evolve from the ones before and always have done. Beliefs change to resolve conflict individually and collectively. As we become aware of alienation from self, aware of alternatives to that, and aware that beliefs are a necessary basis of health, it is time for another change.

A holistic model isn't just a theoretical model; it's a way of being where lifestyle, health and well being are connected with beliefs about self. Belief changes as the higher levels are opened through them having meaning and purpose. Awareness of the transformative vision is spiritual healing. Spiritual healing as awareness of our wholeness and unity is belief that self is an energy field interconnected with environment. This change in awareness has meaning and purpose for our experience and beliefs.

∞

But what about belief in an afterlife? Is that just an optional extra, something we don't want to think about, to be denied or is it of importance to us for the forming of what we are, who we are and believe ourselves to be?

> *Up from Earth's Centre through the seventh gate*
> *I rose and on the Throne of Saturn sate,*
> *And many knots unravelled by the Road*
> *But not the Knot of Human Death and Fate.* (Omar Khayyam; 13th c.)

Omar was a mathematician, astronomer, poet, and Sufi mystic, (Who the potter pray and who the pot?) unitary man in his times, an integration of different pathways. The different paths of knowledge based on reasoning, inspiration based on creativity, belief based on faith and transformation based on meditation are different paths of understanding.

They are similar as using creativity, imagination and reasoning but goals, objectives and possibilities are different. Inspiration is the objective in labs, on stage, on fields, in prayer and ritual, and in moments when time stood still. On the path of transformation the possibilities of self healing are cultural change, prevention of mental illness, and awareness of vision itself. The paths have purpose as the forming of belief as a rational person of science, as a creative artist, or as a person of faith. Belief on the path of transformation forms through a different understanding of what immortality is.

I asked many psychiatrists and psychologists I worked with what mind is, I asked creative people what inspiration is, I asked people of faith what god is, I asked people who practice meditation what the state of meditation is because these issues need to be reflected upon to improve understanding. The answers were mostly different as they were approached from their individual understanding. I never pushed the question, not wanting to be questioning their beliefs as people. The point being that among these educated people there was no common understanding of what these aspects of psyche are. They are not alone; science doesn't know either.

That is understandable because it is difficult to comprehend the unified field because we are part of it; the gold fish in the bowl effect. We become aware of our environment through knowledge based on science, self knowledge gained through experience, beliefs about self and environment and creativity of the imagination.

In his book, **The Transformative Vision,** Arguelles described how architecture, music, painting and literature had lost it's religious function of shaping awareness in medieval society. Any art, lifestyle, beliefs or science that was different was punishable. The 16th century renaissance art movement shaped culture as the function of art was a vision of man as individual. Art became a commercial activity dominated by technique not religious faith. Psyche was then split as the reasoning of technique and creativity of visionary artists. The split shaped culture and that changed history. (p36)

He described creative artists as expressing psyche in their times. They had developed technique and integrated that with their transformative vision of awareness of the self and environment as connected. The outcome was creative art expressing this vision. They captured this on starry nights, as Jerusalem on England's pleasant shores or now as wandering isolated through the streets of London.

Artists expressed what was happening individually and collectively and foreshadowed what needed to change. If the art of expressing psyche's awareness was denied, mankind would not find peace and war would govern the nations.(William Blake). Art is a pathway of understanding that self and environment are connected.

Knowledge is another pathway. As a child I attempted to understand infinity by gazing at the stars and imagining the universe as having no end; did you? I could only know it intuitively. It was an attempt at understanding through knowingness using the imagination not knowledge and as Einstein said, imagination is greater than knowledge because it has limits. He used mental research of visualising everyday examples of how the relationship of gravity, time and space worked. This was not possible using theories that had been established for hundreds of years; that science had limits. Einstein used imagination to establish new theories that he proved mathematically using reasoning.

Knowingness as consciousness is subjective and learnt through experience. Science cannot use reasoning to understand immortality because knowingness is a subjective experience. That does not mean it isn't real, it just can't be measured. I got my feet back on the ground in awareness that infinity can only be experienced as a state of knowingness.

Comprehension that we are energy fields is difficult let alone experiencing it so it has been approached through cultural symbols that are collectively accepted. The symbols and rituals in faiths are different states of consciousness. In Christianity Jesus only asked followers to be remembered as the bread and wine. Their transubstantiation is through the transformation of consciousness as vision. That's how Jesus wanted to be remembered in the ritual.

My understanding of what that state of consciousness was and what was causing it changed my beliefs. I had believed in a personified god, then god as love, god as the unified field being aware of itself, but no longer had belief in a supreme being that is omniscient, omnipotent and omnipresent. Belief changed because of contradictions in that belief. Contradiction were resolved through understanding why awareness changes experience, what spiritual healing is, what the self is as the energy of vision and how we access that energy in meditation and use it as mindfulness in everyday life.

I was visited recently by a friend who is an artist, has had schizophrenia for 18 years and believes that God assisted her recovery. In our talks I told her I no longer believed in a supreme being but that the important thing is that we have beliefs that there is a source of energy but beliefs about what that is and ways of experiencing it are different. I in no way wanted to challenge her belief, the basis of her recovery and resilience as a person. We agreed that experience changes as awareness changes but beliefs about what is causing that are different; she was concerned for my spiritual welfare.

She asked what are my spiritual beliefs if I don't believe in God? I explained there are different paths to understanding... I have belief that self and environment are connected as energy fields. Awareness of that is spiritual healing and we come to this awareness through peace, love and awareness of beauty as the connection of all things. My purpose of writing is to explain what the transformative vision is to make healing accessible to others.

Spiritual beliefs have power when they resolve conflicts. They resolve conflict when they are not about our identity as ego. Spiritual beliefs are intentions to transcend the everyday and in doing so change the experience of it. To be transcendent spiritual beliefs change awareness of what we are and who we are as experience in this life and the next; she was reassured as to my welfare

Awareness, experience, and spiritual beliefs are connected with different ways of being, lifestyle. She agreed with that but said she believed God is love. I do not believe that the energy field is animate; is aware of itself. I believe love is a state of consciousness that opens the 7th level. The difference is belief in what the energy source is. Another level of awareness is opened by the transformative vision of union of all things. I said what matters most is the effect on the brain; she was not aware of neuroplasticity.

She said she has lifestyle goals. I said what you are doing needs to be reframed as goals and objectives of the levels. We sat down together and wrote out her narrative meditation to complement her religious belief; that's what peace as the resolution of differences is.

She contacts me regularly very motivated by goals. They weren't new, but she now had reframed them as understanding of her whole self changed. The list was getting longer. I said to her she was forming a new identity and she was aware of that occurring.

∞

The gods in myths dominated cultures at different times. Cultures resolved the different gods through belief in one god with different aspects. People resolved contradictions in belief in one god through having no religious beliefs, agnosticism or fundamentalism. We resolve them through change in beliefs as we are empowered. Empowerment through awareness of change occurring is well being.

Faith is based on the reasoning of theological interpretations of why experience changes, how we change experience through prayer, and ritual and belief in God as the energy source. The gods are cultural symbols of wholeness of self in awareness of connection with a deity. In mythology gods are omnipresent across time and space. They are power as inspiration in our lives when localised in the present through ritual and prayer that transcends time and place. In that sacred space of consciousness of connection soul is immortal.

In ancient myth, the goddess Gaia was present in sacred groves. In intuitive awareness of connection with nature, she was experienced as inspiration, the mother of all things that is immortal. Psyche in mythology was transformed through her goals of sorting the seeds of awareness, laying bare the golden rams of experience, reaching the goblet of self belief from amidst the raging river Styx, and finally the death of ego in awareness of her own immortality. The gods couldn't do it. Through her tasks she became semi divine; a human with a soul that is immortal. Psyche is identity that is transformed only through our stories.

In identification with the muses, artists are immortal through their creativity. Through their roles as scientists of demonstrating how the universe works, immortality is through the 'holy grail' of knowledge; the highest human potential. There is much wisdom in myths but they need to be useful to our experience in the present. The issue is understanding why belief in an afterlife forms who we are in this life.

Connections occur at different levels of awareness. At the 8th level of awareness of the transformative vision of union all things are connected. Awareness of connection with my environment was experienced where and how I live as dependent on nature for power, water, and growing my trees, through reflection on my experiences as a nurse, through writing, meditation, friends and teachers who existed in the past; in St Francis as service, Buddha as compassion, Mary Magdalene as creativity, Ramana Maharishi as peace, Jesus as unconditional love and Maharishi Yogi as presence. They and others who shared their vision are real to me as energy that inspires. What they inspired was understanding the connection of vision of what the next life is to be with who they were in this life.

I remember them as loving people so ask them in meditation what they would believe about our present times? Reasoning would say that is not possible, but we connect with them as energy of their vision. I believe they would say that transformation is necessary in this life to achieve what the next is to be. Their belief in an afterlife was connected with who they were in this life. This connection was not through the senses or reasoning, but through a knowingness that was difficult to understand. Followers couldn't experience it because it is known only through a change in consciousness as vision.

They were aware that what the afterlife was to be and who they were in the present were connected, so they could not do anything else but live from the inside or be anything else but the self; a state of consciousness of vision. Their vision of the afterlife was who they were in this life which they, except Buddha attributed to belief in a supreme being. He believed that because all phenomena was insubstantial, everything was connected. In this belief reality could be changed through paths of awareness. They were humans but in awareness of soul as immortal they had defeated death. This is what Socrates and they believed, but what is soul?

Soul is a higher level of awareness of self than our individual identity as ego. They as spiritual teachers did not have identity as separate egos. As teachers they were a state of consciousness of awareness of connection of self and self with environment. I believe they were a state of quantum consciousness of vision; that's definitely what a spiritual teacher is. Another characteristic was they were not part of mainstream culture in their times. They in being separate from it allowed them understanding of it. From the mountains and deserts they were teachers that lead us to understanding that soul is the self.

The pathways of reasoning, creativity, and belief are integrated by meditation as a pathway of transformation; the pathway to understanding that soul is our energy field. Is this awareness gained through the separate pathways of science, a celebrity in the different fields, a guru of religious faith, mindfulness of a leaf or different methods of meditation?

A scientist's knowledge is highly specialised, not a generalised way of being. We like to identify with the image of celebrity artists not knowing their whole selves as people. There is something sadder than a theologian without belief, and that is a theologian without self awareness. Mindfulness is a change in consciousness but what is the purpose? The different methods of meditation are different approaches to awareness of self but what is the objective of enlightenment? Narrative Meditation is a method of developing awareness of self to achieve the objective of healing.

How do we as ordinary people gain understanding when the separate paths, having meaning only as for their own sake, result in perception of failure or success that can be fleeting. Material success can be fleeting 'like snowflakes on the dusty desert sands, in a moment they are gone' (Omar Khayyam) because of identity as ego. Surrender of that is not giving up. Surrender of ego occurs through the transformation of awareness, experience and belief.

A friend practices yoga and meditation is part of that. Yoga is a path of change in awareness and experience through the connection of mind, body and spirit. Yoga means union, but what are beliefs about that? She had the experience of the state of meditation but not the understanding of what it was. She asked me to explain it because she was happy with this new level of awareness.

I explained it as the transformative vision where there is no time or objects; she remembered it as that state. She asked how did I understand her experience? I explained access to the transformative vision is possible on paths of understanding. We may access it but need to understand that experience as having meaning and purpose. There will be more questions as she remembers her experience and goals form as a meditation on healing.

She rand me a month later and said life was a 'blast'. She had found a job she really liked, gave her more money, time and because she had more time had new inspiration as an artist, and had found a creative community where she would like to live; all the events had happened coincidentally. We talked about why mindfulness of goals changes experience. She said it's wonderful and I should talk to more people about it. I said that's what I do as my source of inspiration. Perhaps I need to integrate technique and creativity with a medium of connecting with others.

Coping, resilience is problem solving, adjusting response to problems that can't be resolved and maintaining a generalised state of physical and mental well being. Meditation is about acquiring all three skills to prevent ego's problem of alienation; a state of absence of awareness of connection of self and self with environment. Not wanting that is when an alternative belief that self and environment are connected begins to take form.

Narrative Meditation as an internal technology of change is an integration; an integration of the reasoning of physics that the universe is an energy field, neuroscience that brain changes structure and functioning as awareness changes, holism as the personal art of living, and belief that self and environment are a unified energy field. The practice is to awareness of our wholeness and unity and a wise person once said to pray constantly in silence. Meditation is our silent prayer on what is sacred within. Mindfulness makes the prayer constant. The afterlife is a given but what it is to be, I attribute to meditation and belief in spirituality. Belief that soul is our energy field forms what and who we are in this life and the next.

For Omar in 13th century, the seventh level did not resolve the question of death and destiny in life. In resolving the question of what the afterlife is to be, the question is resolved. The self to be a transcendent state of consciousness must transcend our own mortality. There is existence after death. The afterlife is the energy of consciousness. Reincarnation is consciousness reforming as matter; what we believe ourselves to be. The afterlife is unravelled through belief in what we are.

Consciousness creates our reality of experience in this life individually and collectively. The self is state of consciousness of vision of what the afterlife is to be; a state of synchronicity of consciousness and experience. This vision of the afterlife, is what we are as the self in this life. In meditation and in mindfulness of this objective we are the self. On the path of transformation, belief in what the afterlife is to be forms what and who we are as experience in this life.

The aspect of belief is changing in awareness that soul is our energy field that is eternal as the self; the sixth possibility of vision.

∞

Spiritual healing is a process of transformation of awareness as mindfulness in everyday life, experience as healing, and spirituality as belief that connects them. Spirituality is belief that the energy field is individual, between us and a universal unified field, that consciousness is our energy field, that what we are as energy and believe ourselves to be is who we are as experience. The pyramid is symbolic of the self as energy that is eternal.

∞

The inner journey is to awareness of the transformative vision of union of self with environment. The outer journey is remembering vision as experience changes. The aspects of experience of body, emotions, thoughts and belief connect at the apex through their transformation as service, compassion, creativity, and spirituality. Awareness of what we are as energy and believe ourselves to be is who we are as experience. Spirituality as belief connects awareness and experience.

The transformative vision of awareness of union with the energy field is a state of consciousness of vision. Awareness, experience and belief have been transforming as mirrors of vision. Mindfulness of principles, goals, and objectives is vision in everyday life. We are made whole as a mirror of the energy of vision because of neuroplasticity of the brain. Vision as energy is a state of quantum consciousness that is causing this to occur.

As we remember the transformative vision our framework is transforming as a mirror of consciousness. Change is occurring as connections are made. Awareness and experience are connected by belief but what connects them?

Identity

A beginning practitioner mental health nurse gains knowledge. However you need more than science to assist others and science does change. You need awareness of self and a method of change to assist healing. The therapeutic outcome for others is well being. The therapeutic use of self is an objective and the integration of values, awareness, experience and beliefs about self. Integrating them is the art of practice of an expert nurse.

The forming of identity is the firm ground on which to stand in circumstances that are changing. Awareness of self develops to assist others with health crises. The expert nurse is a state of consciousness of mindfulness of goals and objectives. As a practicing nurse I used care planning as a method of change. My practice was changing my identity as an expert nurse and the identity of patients as people.

One lady with schizophrenia for over 20 years told me that participating in her care plan with me was the best therapy she had ever had. What is the evidence base of psychotherapies if they don't consider neuroplasticity of the brain? The method is an intervention based on patient goals and objectives and review of outcomes of experience; objective, subjective and team assessment of progress towards objectives.

She was not a patient identified as her diagnosis and stigmatised because of that throughout her life. In becoming aware of her own strengths, her identity had changed as a person. She was not just a patient of Female One, Room 6, Bed 9. Recovery from mental health crises is about empowerment through using our strengths. What is recovered is identity.

I care coordinated a patient who had treatment resistant schizophrenia, had a physical illness which prevented him being prescribed newer, more effective medications, a history of crime, suicide attempts and violence in response to auditory hallucinations; my role was looking after high dependency patients by developing a therapeutic alliance.

We discussed his belief that his phantom arm was connected with the stars which were the souls of the deceased which explained to him where his voices came from. This was confirmed to him by his understanding of Egyptian mythology (!) He believed that on his passing he became a star just like a pharaoh. What would you say to him? Now of course amputees are educated to tell their brains that their limbs are no longer there. I would take that into my meditation as a service to my body to remember that. Meditation changes if circumstances change.

I said that is a beautiful thought as stars are symbols of connection with the universe; he agreed with that. Lack of abstract thinking is a symptom of schizophrenia and is absence of awareness of self the cause? I escorted him to visit his mother who lived in another state. He had lost contact with her for many years, so we stayed for a few nights. The visit went well until he looked anxious and excused himself from the dinner table. He explained to me he had 'seen' his mother form beautiful angelic wings. I reassured him that it was just a beautiful image of his mother and he was ok with that.

Intentionally imagining something is different from the experience in schizophrenia of visual hallucinations which are not controlled. I made sure he took his PRN meds before going off to bed; he slept well. His mother enjoyed the experience and he did as well.

The therapeutic use of self is learnt through experiences. Reasoning is why, how, and what needs to occur. The art of practice is putting it all together. It's all about service, compassion, and creativity knowing what the objective are in the present moment; reconnecting a mother and son.

Identity forms through awareness of values, principles, goals and objectives for self and others. Integrating them is the art of how things are done and that's the process of change in identity as an expert nurse. Nurses worked in my services as transformative therapists using self and care planning as a method of change. But it may not be a decision to identify as the self but many believed nursing had a sacred function. In mental health nursing the sacred function was the therapeutic use of self to restore identity as empowered individuals and prevent mental health crises reoccurring.

As a nurse the self is awareness of body, emotions, thoughts, and beliefs. Awareness changes through meditation on the levels. This change in awareness changes psyche, our identity of who we are.

∞

I had an experience of meditation in 1967. It was through a guru, Maharishi Yogi but I did not understand it. I had the experience of meditation but not the understanding to enable me to remember that experience again. Gurus inspire meditation however he explained it from his level of awareness, how he learnt it, his experience, and culture of customs and beliefs which may or may not be helpful to our understanding at the time.

Cultural beliefs are different philosophies, faiths and ways of being but what connects non duality of Hinduism, Zen Buddhism, Taoism, Sufism, western mysticism, spirituality and Celtic connection with nature (the pipes still call to me) is the self. The approaches are based on history, culture, customs, practices, and knowledge but the objective of realisation of the self is the same.

Just being in the presence of a guru is a meditation. Gurus inspire meditation as we connect with their energy. Their energy is total awareness of goals and objectives in the present moment. A guru's state of connection with this energy inspires a state of meditation in others. I thought of it then as a state of Zen, a state of connection with environment. But then I wondered what is the purpose of this altered state of consciousness, why should we want to change everything was ok for me, I was healthy, the cold war was stalemated as a balance of terror, we were shooting for the moon, the times were changing lifestyles, conscription was a few years away, and the antiwar movement was gathering strength, there were pizzas, many great learning experiences, work, technology and music was inspiring Friday on our minds; there was hope for the future but vision was not yet remembered; to me it had no purpose.

The alternative lifestyle movement in the 60's was analysed as a crisis of adolescence; what crisis? It was awareness of problems in the present, hope of a better lifestyle and awareness that we were heading for a crisis in the future if things didn't change. Collectively we were still adolescents; identity was still forming. It was all about interpretation of what free love is, understanding of issues, and how they could be changed.

The solution to this was the opening of the doors of perception through drugs. Perception is not the same thing as reality. The doors are opened by understanding that what is inside is the self. The self wasn't remembered because cultures change slowly, technology was improving and lifestyle in the city looked better than life on the rural commune with its problems. Interestingly technological change, outer and inner is assisting with those problems making lifestyle change viable and a now a desirable if not even a necessary lifestyle option.

As I remembered the experience of meditation much later, I was the self in awareness that the guru was the self. That's what the meditation was. You can leave the place but not understanding that experience. The different methods of meditation are states of connection with the self. The quest is understanding what the self is and how we access and use it. As I remember, the quest never ended; that's what gurus do, they inspire a quest of understanding.

The learning experience is understanding why meditation as a neuroplastic exercise is changing experience, what the self is as a state of quantum consciousness, and how we access that energy through the transformative vision and use it in everyday life. Knowledge that we are energy fields is the most profound thought and challenging. The challenge is to use this energy through mindfulness of goals to change experience if needed. That's what empowerment is all about.

∞

When I finished a draft of this book, I realised how my three books were connected. It's not easy to write but is my source of inspiration that guides me. Connecting them now was inspirational for me as a guide, a writer and as a person.

I was writing from my level of awareness of self. Ego is a state of alienation from connection with self, others and environment. **Do you Remember** was ego on an inner journey of learning meditation. It was about how through remembering experience in my roles, and meditation awareness of self develops. The ending of the inner journey was remembering the archetypal image of wholeness and unity, the transformative vision. **As We Remember** was about how through remembering the transformative vision on the outer journey, consciousness is changing experience as through the forming of goals. **Remembering of the Self** started as how belief forms...

I believed my three books were about self healing. I was aware of how they followed one another as awareness, experience and belief but not aware of another story evolving through them; a narrative of change in awareness of what we are, who we are, and believe ourselves to be; the narrative of remembering the self.

Psyche is awareness of what and who we are; identity. As a nurse the self is body, emotions, thoughts, and beliefs. Through experience and meditation psyche's transformation is the connection of our framework of awareness, experience, and beliefs. Identity as ego is the integration of consciousness, experience as outcome of cause and effect and belief in man as matter only; but we intuitively know we are more than that; our identity as ego is fake.

Meditation develops awareness of our whole self as our goals and objectives. Our whole self is an energy field. Our whole self is our framework of awareness, experience, and beliefs connected. What is transforming them as possibilities is vision. The parts are connected through their transformation as mirrors of vision. The self is state of consciousness of vision. Our parts are connected by belief in identity as the self. Identity as the self is their connection. The narrative is psyche's transformation of identity. The pyramid is symbolic of identity as the self.

Narrative Meditation is a method of change and transformation through self healing. The method of change is transforming our framework as an integrated whole. The transformation of identity as ego is occurring as we spiritually heal. Mastery is a lifestyle decision of how to be is made in awareness of possibilities of vision of transformation of awareness as mindfulness of goals in everyday life, experience as individual, transpersonal and spiritual healing, and belief as spirituality. What we are as energy, who we are as experience, and believe ourselves to be form identity. Psyche is only transformed through stories. The self can only be remembered through our own stories of transformation. Through understanding what the self is as energy, and how we access that through the transformative vision and use it, the self is remembered.

∞

As a guide this book is about how the self is remembered. My understanding of meditation and the third stage changed. The self is state of consciousness of vision. Vision is healing the levels and transforming our framework as an integrated whole. It is the energy of vision that has been opening the levels. In mindfulness of all principles, goals, and objectives ego is transformed. As a guide this book is about how the self can be remembered as an intention. Meditation changes as understanding changes. I changed my meditation.

At the 8th level the goal is the transformative vision of union, the objective of spiritual healing is identity as the self. The transformative vision and identity are connected, giving meditation on the 8th level new meaning and purpose. The transformative vision has meaning as union and purpose as the transformation of identity. In meditation on the transformative vision of the unified field of there being no time or objects identity is the self. The aspect of belief is fully formed as belief in identity as the self; the seventh possibility of vision.

∞

The decision is made in awareness of possibilities but what difference does a decision make? As a nurse the decision of how to practice is a decision to identify as an expert nurse. It may not be a decision to identify as the self or how to be. In understanding of what the self is as energy and how we access and use it, the decision of how to be is a choice.

The decision of how to be is a decision to identify as the self. Mastery of Narrative Meditation is belief in identity as the self and a lifestyle decision of how to be made in awareness of the possibility of psyches transformation as the self. The possibility of transformation of what I am, who I am and believe myself to be. Mastery is a way of being as a person.

The levels of meditation are different levels of healing as an individual, transpersonal and spiritual being. Spiritual healing is belief in identity as the self. As experience identity as the self is awareness that vision is the energy of our whole selves and using it to self heal. Identity as the self is a state of synchronicity of vision, inner experience of healing of the levels, transformation of the outer aspects and outer serendipitous events that assist us realise goals and objectives. It occurs as we move into the universal energy field through the decision.

We are energy fields. Awareness of that is transforming experience, beliefs and identity. The decision acknowledges meditation as a method of transformation. As we remember what we are through regular practice the inner and outer are connected. The decision grounds self in this new reality; a new beginning of experience.

The method is a neuroplastic exercise of using vision to self heal. Access to the transformative vision is not to be an onlooker. In the state of meditation we are not an observer but the self. The decision is psyche's movement into the unified field. In myth Psyche became semi divine; a human with a soul that is immortal. Through the decision we give direction to our energy field in this life and the next. The decision is identification with that which is eternal; the self.

Awareness of the self is the end of the quest of understanding that leaves just a decision to be made if mastery is an objective. It is made in awareness of a crisis affecting most people in different ways and awareness of possibilities as alternatives to that. As a nurse awareness of self develops to assist others. Recovery from mental health crises is about empowerment using our strengths. What is recovered is identity. My role as a manager was about analysis of trends to prevent crises occurring. The decision is made in awareness of a collective crisis of consciousness to be of service in our circumstances.

∞

It is said we all have our own individual inner reality. In identity as ego that is true but it is only partially true. Awareness of what and who we are, our identity is formed within our culture of collective beliefs and behaviours; there are differences in circumstances. There are two different realities based on our awareness, experience, and beliefs. One is known through cause and effect of reasoning which science uses to explain it and develop technologies from it which are useful for daily living. A different reality based on synchronicity exists simultaneously with it in the present. This becomes known using an internal technology of change which is also useful for daily living.

Existing in the paradox is the sum of human experience and probably has always been since our cultural mythic time in the garden of dreams. Myths of our cultures become relevant when understanding of them resolves differences of time, place, belief and identity. What resolves these differences is vision. A different reality is experienced through vision being remembered in the present, individually and collectively.

I had finished my last book coincidentally on the same day Donald Trump was elected President. I thought about the significance of that for understanding of the importance of culture. To me it highlighted a difference with collective awareness of what and who we are in the present. America's history of industrial strength was the issue when the age of iron has definitely past. The American dream of happiness as materiality is passing but vision of a better future is not.

The collective crisis is a state of consciousness where there is no connection of self, and self with environment at a higher level of awareness. The election was a symptom of a crisis without vision being actualised through reasoning of policies based on values and principles, a system of responsibility and accountability for that and hope of a better future; what really made the USA great.

Where identity is ego, self image is our roles. Without reasoning, a method of change, and vision of the future ego doesn't cope with complexity, diversity, or has the ability to see what change is needed, and in increasing denial of the crisis, resorts to blaming and control as solutions. The event underlies the importance of vision to integrate self, people, states and nations; what the founders believed in. It was about diversity succeeding using a system of democracy to achieve the vision of a better future for all at home and even abroad.

Ego is a state of consciousness of division of self and self from environment. Our reality of experience is a mirror of identity. Where there is no connection at higher level of awareness, the crisis of consciousness is a crisis of identity as ego. Alienation is a symptom of loss of awareness of self.

The trump hand of ego is power to control of the reality of experience of others. Power is control through division that creates conflict within self and between others and doing whatever it takes to achieve that becomes the norm. The control of the reality of experience is normalising that war is peace, love is hate speech, equality is lower taxes for the wealthy, opportunity is closing services, democracy is freedom to manipulate, and loyalty is accepting these as true. What ego doesn't understand is there are greater causes than themselves to serve.

Ego in it's drive for control is not aware of self or concerned for the experience of others. The risk is fear leading to anger causing more division. Fear and anger are traps that further divide self and self from others. Just around the corner is descent into a self fulfilling vortex of more use of power if we are not inspired by a different way. I am inspired by the vision of Gandhi, Mandela, and King who dared to share a dream of collective change occurring through peace and love; in working for them can also work for us individually and collectively. Black lives also matter.

Material man is a state of consciousness of identity as ego. Who we are is our roles, living in a material universe governed by physics, motivated by self interest and relying on the external technologies of science to fix all the problems. The crisis of consciousness is a crisis of identity. The crisis is a state of alienation from awareness of connection with our whole selves, and our material, social, and natural environment and we are becoming aware of that through trends and crises over the past 30 years.

What we get when there is no awareness of principles of service, compassion, creativity, peace, love, beauty, connection of self with environment and others is a state of alienation, absence of belief in our connection. Ego is a state of alienation and self interest is the only governing principle. That's the illogic of identity as ego. The crisis of consciousness is alienation from self and there are different symptoms of it.

What we get is increasing climate change, domestic and other violence, terrorism, organised crime, war, GFC, and addictions as symptoms of alienation from self, others, community and society caused by identity as ego. Mental illnesses are increasing as a symptom of a crisis of alienation from self. Yet we wonder why these events and trends are happening when the problem lies within.

Societies are dominated by social institutions of religion that control morality, political parties who control laws and multinationals who control the economy and information. They can't assist change because they are based on short term corporate self interest. The crisis in challenging the well being of self and others, challenges our identity as individuals.

I know I talk too much to others about the weather, they say it's a sign of aging but it's not just me. The local news predicts this year there will be more than average numbers of storms, drought, heatwaves, bushfires, cyclones, and that the Great Barrier Reef is under increasing threat. The UN has just stated that there needs to be zero greenhouse gas emissions by 2050 to prevent a catastrophic climate shift; Al Gore agrees and predicts that as a possible threat to civilisation as we know it. Many others are becoming concerned about it and are aware of other problems with our social, economic, and natural environment as effects of our culture of materialism.

Climate is in a more rapid state of change. This changes our awareness of the connection of the well being with the broader environment and culture. People do think globally and act locally but generally the effect is disempowerment experienced as perplexity, concern for the future or denial expressing as the blaming of others.

Ego is a cultural identity that defines us as our roles that are changing as never before. The crisis is a collapsing of ego from within and the problem affects everyone in different ways. The crisis is resolved in awareness of what it is and through our empowerment. Change can only come as individuals are empowered through their own transformation. Awareness of the connection of individual well being with wider events and trends and culture of material self interest is known through reasoning and intuition, a change in awareness that is shared between many who hope for signs of change.

A hopeful sign is that millennials are more aware, have greater opportunities through access to knowledge and skills, are mobile and can articulate their concerns but need a sense of purpose, a spark of inspiration to ignite hope for a better future. The problem is an opportunity to redefine what and who they want to be using an internal technology of change. In virtual reality the observer is a passive recipient of images created by someone else. The transformative vision is accessed by using our own imagination. The hope is psyches transformation.

Each stage of the development of a civilisation is however based on change in collective cultural beliefs. Culture shape consciousness and who we are as individuals. Individual change in awareness is a wider change in awareness happening. Individually we heal as an intention in awareness of the transformative vision; a change in consciousness. As that develops a renaissance of culture is the outcome that changes collective awareness and experience.

Cultures shape us as individuals and in turn is being shaped by individuals because change in awareness causes neuroplastic changes and always has done. Cultures as collective beliefs and behaviours are slow movements but as we change the world as our circumstances changes and we are aware of that occurring. The cycle of transformation is occurring as we individually heal. That's what the present times are, a time of individual transformation between ages. The ages were changes in technologies that changed awareness, experience, and beliefs. A new civilisation began through their integration.

How can we assist this in our circumstances now? The solution isn't to reopen psychiatric hospitals; with control as the agenda they are prisons with doctors run by a controlling nurse; get the picture of how places of safety become nests of control? What we need is to become part of the solution by;

- Maintaining and improving our own well being
- Living as service to others and environment through finding creative solutions to problems
- Joining groups with shared values and objectives of change in attitudes and behaviour
- In awareness of self as ego, identity is our roles. In awareness of identity as the self we get on with our roles but it is the art of how we do them that makes all the difference.

People who are creative and in roles as artists need to use their creative skills to step up to a social function through supporting what is right and not supporting what isn't. Creativity denied is a denial of psyche's awareness of the present and hope for the future. When psyche isn't expressed there is no creativity. Without it all art as technique and style are commodities. The task is to make a living from being authentic creative visionaries.

Arguelles wrote that the transformative vision is awareness of connection of self and environment. Psyche is expressing this awareness through creative artists. My understanding of the transformative vision how it develops, its meaning and purpose is different. The difference is reasoning that awareness of connection is developing in our times through understanding the transformative vision of union, the state of meditation. As we remember the transformative vision psyche is transformed to heal. That's the purpose of the art of meditation.

Psyche is transforming to connect self and self with environment in our present times to maintain well being. Why is this important for artists now? Psyche is a broad canvas. The canvas is the energy field on which forms of art express what we are aware of ourselves as being. Which paths we use to express psyche are individual but psyche's transformation is only through our stories however that is expressed. For me now as a guide I write about the story of psyche's transformation. Psyche takes form as the self but the separate paths connected as a culture change history. That's what a renaissance is all about.

∞

Arguelles as a visionary wrote in 1975; 'Yet today, from pole to pole the world shakes; a presence long silent moves again; a form unseen, but not unfelt; a name unvoiced, but not unknown.'(p15). Psyche is being shaped through experience individually and collectively in the present; what is being shaken is awareness, what is being felt is the energy field, and the name unvoiced but not yet remembered is the self. Our transformation occurs through belief in identity as the self.

∞

The coincidence highlighted to me opposites of the book being about the self and vision of a future achieved through empowerment, while the election was about ego and control through division. It highlighted the inner work to be done in the present and the need to assist change in our circumstances.

Psyche can be likened to the solitary joker as the game unfolds and aware now of what the game is all about wins through its power to transform. We become aware of what we are through remembering the playing of hands and what the stakes are. The possible risk of not fulfilling our potential is that consciousness can be shaped in the interest of others if we don't have the firm ground of identity on which to stand.

In the 70s I read **1984** by the visionary George Orwell. I read it as an ominous prediction of a society controlled by coercion. I read it without understanding how the technology of 'big brother' controlled individual consciousness. It was controlled through rewriting history, changing the language and 'doublethink', a statement containing two opposites that created conflict within self. The only resolution of this conflict was love of big brother. The ominous part was the society was not aware of this happening. I now understood why reality TV programs are popular! Viewers vicariously identify with the power of control of the reality of experience of others!

Authoritarianism means control of consciousness through coercion and consent. A digital dictatorship takes big brother a step closer. (ABC Foreign Correspondent; 18. 09.18). People in believing that is necessary to control criminal behaviour and advance through social credits have made the bargain. You do not agree to the bargain if you believe in individual rights and don't like the thought of entering Room 101! Room 101 is a metaphor of alienation from the self.

Marshal McLuhan wrote that the technology of the media, the medium is the message that changes individual identity as consumers of products and services and in doing so changes societies. He wrote that before the internet was invented and neuroplasticity was understood. The web in connecting us at many levels as individuals, communities, societies, cultures, and as economies changes our awareness.

The technology in making connections shrinks the world as a global village which has benefits in some ways depending on how it is used. There are risks of the medium if we don't have the firm ground of individual and collective identity on which to stand. Google Cambridge Analytica for understanding how the technology can also be used to give messages to exploit fears and change voting behaviour without anyone being aware of that occurring.

History can also be changed when nobody knows what policies mean, what was said was meant and trust in institutions that analyse news and administer justice is undermined, (Insert a very sad faced emoji). We are fortunate in being better educated can critically analyse doublethink that war is peace, freedom is slavery, ignorance is strength and even that more assault rifles means safety. We need to think about the importance of education for critical and creative thinking and for the understanding of history.

Every abomination in history was caused by the pursuit of power by egotistic individuals, regardless of religious creed, ideological dogma or political colour of their group; they were just means to an end. The fact that they caused enormous suffering to others, theirs, others societies and environment did not matter; it's was only about power for it's own sake. Education is about awareness of the past to critically analyse the present so as not to repeat that in the future. That's what global sanity is.

∞

Our transformation occurs through understanding meditation as the art of the remembering of the self. Through practicing it the self can be remembered as an intention. Our transformation is necessary for a change in collective awareness and experience to happen. Through individual transformation a renaissance of culture occurs through education based on science, the arts based on creativity, belief based on spirituality and their integration using meditation as the art of transformation. They become pillars of a renewed society because they bring about change in collective awareness and experience and we are aware of that occurring.

The decision is made in awareness of a collective crisis of consciousness, what that is as a crisis of identity, awareness of possibilities as alternatives to that, understanding why our individual transformation is important for a change in culture, and how we can be of service in our circumstances.

Connected

Scientists debate whether the pyramids of Giza were tombs or religious centres; I believe they were spiritual healing centres. The purpose of the pyramids is change in awareness through understanding them. They were not temples you go inside, you go inside yourself to heal. As healing centres they changed awareness. They were placed to mirror Orion, the birthplace of stars in relation to the Milky Way as the Nile, the source of temporal life and the sphinx rising gazing from the sands at eternal life. The structures were placed in belief that the celestial universe, the temporal, and afterlife were connected. As healing centres awareness of them and environment as connected changed experience in this life and the next.

They had vision of what the afterlife was to be. A 2,500 year old sarcophagus of a priestess was recently opened by accident at Sydney University and had her name and an inscription;

Mer-Neith-it-es

"Speak my name so I may live again"

She believed in her vision of what the afterlife was to be which made her who she was in life; that's what identity as a priestess is. As tombs they symbolised the power of the pharaoh that lay within. The pharaoh's power was vision that building the pyramids was important then and for the future. The pyramid is symbol of the self within that in awareness of connection with its environment is immortal. The pharaoh on passing became a star in the heavens.

As symbols of the self the pyramid is an interconnected whole, built level upon level. The pyramid is an integration of its framework of foundations, the levels, the aspects and apex where they all meet. The structures became spiritual healing centres through understanding them as symbols of the self as whole in awareness of the universal, the temporal and afterlife as connected. Understanding that is a change in the individuals framework of awareness, experience, belief and identity. The pyramids are a plan of our framework that changes as understanding changes. The pharaoh's power of vision unified the civilisation through its culture; that's what a pharaoh does.

As healing centres the pyramid transforms as a symbol of the self; a quest that crosses all of time. Healing occurs through understanding them; that is why we are still mysteriously drawn to them. Understanding why awareness changes experience, what the self is as the energy of vision and how we access and use it, gives meditation on the pyramid meaning and purpose.

The pyramid is a symbol of our framework of parts. At the apex of awareness identity as the self is their connection. The pyramid is symbol of the self as the energy of consciousness that makes us whole. It is made whole as our unconscious energy field becomes known in awareness of the transformative vision. Narrative Meditation can be understood as a method of change through self healing and transformation of our framework. Identity forms in awareness of the possibility of the self as eternal. Like the meaning of the pyramids as healing centres, identity as the self has only been forgotten.

Understanding of the meaning and purpose of the pyramid changes as awareness, experience, and belief changes. The pyramid has changed in meaning as a symbol; of ourselves as levels of awareness, of the unconscious image of unity of self and environment that makes us whole, of our energy field as this whole self, of our framework of awareness, experience, and belief, of the self as a state of quantum consciousness of vision, of the self as energy that is eternal, and purpose as how we remember the self. Construction the pyramid of awareness, and the transformation of psyche are connected.

∞

I asked myself who would connect with this meditation? I think like me, there are many interested in the possibilities of mind. People interested in neuroscience that the brain is plastic, what that means for meditation as a neuroplastic exercise, and what that means for health, well being and happiness as our reality of experience. Meditation is a method of self healing to maximise our potential. How we do that is using Narrative Meditation as our internal technology of change and transformation.

People in the 'pre contemplation' stage who are unsure of why or how to practice and what the possible benefits are. People who have physical, emotional, or psychological issues for who the medical model of treating problems is not working and are willing to trial a holistic approach. The approach is using meditation as a neuroplastic exercise of using strengths of reasoning and creativity.

Fortunate people who have no issues but are aware that life involves stress, stress accumulates and becomes free floating, we don't want that and that meditation is preventative of stress. People who want to experience their fullest potential and who doesn't want that? Beginners who want to experience meditation more deeply. People involved in service to others as health workers and carers. Self healing is necessary in vocations of service to maintain well being. We need to refresh by hitting the reboot button at times to go back inside to the sacred space within.

Researchers who are interested in our potential to self heal. Deepak Chopra developed the idea of quantum healing occurring as mind corrects disease in the body.(**Quantum Healing**, p. 257). Scientists do not know if there are any links between quantum consciousness acquired through meditation and cellular change and may never know. To science the unified energy field will only exist if it can be reduced to a mathematical equation. As a subjective state of consciousness and experience it cannot be understood by scientists.

We are energy fields. Vision is energy when it changes our experience through self healing. I am not aware of all the possibilities of self healing using the method and for science to find out. Understanding the method makes research possible into the benefits of maximising our potential. With research it could be used as complementary to treatment. A very different holistic practice would develop through the integration of meditation with treatment. There are social, economic, and humanitarian incentives of using meditation to assist prevent lifestyle related diseases, to recover from the different types of trauma, and to maximise our potential.

People who like me believe that a renaissance is necessary. Our culture is almost completely dominated by corporations whose business is to shape our awareness as consumers of their products and services. In doing so they shape identity and inadvertently create our reality of experience; that's the way it is but we can modify that.

We may know change is necessary but wonder if that involves the sacrifice of gains. The sacrifice to be made is identity as ego. We are individuals interconnected with our environment. Awareness of that and what individually to do about it is no sacrifice at all; it's an opportunity to develop our full potential.

A renaissance is necessary to develop our fullest potential for control of our destiny and well being. A renaissance has pillars of education, the arts, meditation as the art of living, and belief based on spirituality. A renaissance occurs through our transformation. Narrative Meditation is a method of individual and collective transformation.

People interested in the prevention of mental illness and we all should be. Cultural beliefs that define our individual boundaries as ego, determine what and who we are as experience. Psychoanalysis said ego is necessary as our boundaries of self and environment and that mental illness is its blurring. Our boundaries of who we are and is necessary but identity as ego isn't.

Our boundaries are not physical. They are formed through principles, goals and objectives. Our boundaries are consciousness that changes as we become self aware. Grounded in awareness of what and who we are is well being. Mental illnesses are a symptom of a collective crisis of consciousness of identity. That mental illness is a collective crisis of identity wasn't obvious in the past; a very few thinkers thought it was. It was always attributed to genetics and biochemistry that can be treated. Defined as a symptom of a collective crisis the focus needs to shift to prevention.

Accessing mental health services has increased over the past decade and continues to rise. As services they are responsible for treatment, and rehabilitation; not prevention. Education is the basis of prevention. Mindfulness training has started as part of school curricula to help prevent the one in seven primary school children and thirty percent increase in young people experiencing mental illness. Increasing levels of suicide in a society is a symptom of a collective crisis.

Narrative meditation is a method of development of awareness to achieve health, happiness and well being to maximise our potential and in doing so prevent mental health crises occurring. Mental illness is prevented through empowerment in awareness of change occurring and identity as what we are, who we are and believe ourselves to be forms.

In awareness of meditation as a neuroplastic exercise it could be used as part of the recovery plan through integration of rehabilitation goals with it. If relapse occurs, people know how to return to health through goals as the firm ground on which we stand and in doing so recover identity. We recover from any tragic loss using our strengths. We need in times of loss to find new ways of how to be; that's what transformation is all about, individually and collectively.

People who practice awareness of the chakras as a meditation, believe they as states of consciousness are energy, believe our whole self is an energy field, wonder what the possibilities of full consciousness are, believe in an afterlife and wonder if that, their experience and their practice are connected.

The levels as energy need to be refreshed to remain dynamic; they are never static as so to speak. They are refreshed by principles that give them new meaning and goals and objectives that give them purpose as our circumstances change; and they are. Our transformation occurs through their merging; another level of awareness is opened through vision.

Knowledge that this method is a neuroplastic exercise refreshes the levels to open up new possibilities. Vision of what the afterlife is to be, is what we are as the self in this life. The 8th level has meaning as union and purpose as the transformation of identity as the self that is eternal.

People who practice meditation through music, and mantras. I had used the seven notes of the scale linked with mantras as a meditation. They were effective in tuning my whole self but what was the purpose of this for experience, what are beliefs about that, and what did it have to do with identity? The 7th level mantra OM needs a key change to the octave of union; the sound of silence of the 8th level. We need new approaches and techniques of meditation that have purpose as healing as the sound of the transformative vision is planted. It is planted through understanding what it is, and how we access and use it.

People who do have a vision of well being, want a lifestyle that is consistent with values and maximises their potential but wonder about what the holistic mix is, how to achieve it, and what are beliefs about it? The vision is achieved through meditation on goals. Belief changes as the higher levels have meaning as individual, transpersonal, and spiritual healing and purpose as the remembering of the self.

People who are reflective, creative, may or may not believe in a supreme being but believe there is an energy source but don't yet believe that consciousness is that source. People interested in spirituality. The interest is triggered by a collective movement of awareness that individual well being and environment are connected. Spirituality is not an organised religion or a cult. A cult's objective is to isolate the individual to control identity as member of that group while spirituality is the forming of individual identity through awareness of connection with others and our whole environment.

Aesthetics who are inspired by beauty, when time and place are transcended. Those moments of connection with environment are real and experienced in meditation as the beauty of the opening of the levels. The inspiration that the self is a field of energy is a very beautiful thought.

People who aspire to the possibility of living from the inside but unsure what that means and what is its purpose? It is a shift from being blown by the winds of the external. This possibility is learnt, building upon self healing, renaissance, prevention of mental illness and vision achieving a transformation of awareness, experience, and belief. To be empowered is to live from the inside.

We are empowered by knowing that the truth behind our experience is our transformation. The truth is seen and felt when the knower believes that identity as the self is the firm ground on which to stand to create our experience in the present. We were entertained by the movie, **Avatar**. We can also relate to the narrative of the hero as our own transformation quest. In a state of connection with the planet the star connected with their energy source of peace, love and beauty, transforming his identity and experience.

The journey of reasoning, creativity, faith and meditation is shared by many. The vision quest however is individual, because our culture doesn't support a quest of finding out what and who we are. When vision is collectively forgotten, the quest has no meaning or purpose. The journey is about understanding what the self is. The quest is the transformation of identity as the self; the star within.

∞

Songs about the beauty of connection are expressions of the self. Through poems, prayers, promises and things that we believe in we can find a better way. I was put in two minds by a song. I liked the music and the lyrics that soul was free, we were star dust and golden and needed to get ourselves back to the garden but I did not understand what soul or the garden was let alone how to get back to it. Identity changes in retreat in the garden of the self.

In mythology, Eden was a garden of inspiration where everything was created. We weren't cast from it; it wasn't a place but the space of consciousness of connection with environment. We weren't ejected but forgot the self as identity changed. Change can only occur if we accept responsibility and know how to return. The garden of the self was only forgotten and we get back into it in awareness of why we left and as we remember the self we return.

We go back into it in meditation on the self, and stay in it through mindfulness in everyday life. The garden of the self is a state of vision, of mindfulness of goals and objectives where we create our experience in the present moment. As we individually remember, the great return is a renaissance of culture that is the connection of the pillars.

∞

People who wonder about the why, how and the what of the Great Pyramid. This book is about understanding what a pyramid is all about. Constructing it is the integration of body, mind and identity as psyche's quest of transformation.

Finally people who are interested in the possibility of living in the present moment but wonder what that means and how. Where the past and future meet is the present moment. What is living in the present moment?

The transformative vision is the past, and future meeting. In awareness of union there is no past or future only the eternal now; that's what the transformative vision of the unified field is. Living in the present moment is a state of consciousness of all things as connected at a higher level of awareness of vision.

I know what you are thinking; living in the present moment is the eighth possibility but that would be a wrong conclusion. It's not a possibility of vision; it's what vision is. This could lead to an interesting after dinner discussion or to a new way of being.

Awareness that there are many approaching or already on the path of transformation is realisation that there are many who would connect with this meditation. Through constructing the pyramid we construct our lives. We can work through experience one block at a time which is hard work or through understanding the transformative vision the work is made a lot easier. That's how all pyramids are built.

The pyramid and life are connected. They are connected as understanding changes. The conclusion of this book is how understanding the meaning and purpose of the transformative vision leads to the state of meditation and healing.

There is another reason; journeys end sometime; that's the quest.

Conclusion

I started writing this book as a final chapter and conclusion that should have been after a friend asked me how do we use vision in everyday life? That inspired me to think that knowledge that we are an energy field must be of use to us in daily living; that inspiration lead to this book.

I went into the garden of the self and asked have I achieved my objectives as a guide, a writer and as a person? As a guide this book is about the method of Narrative Meditation. As a meditation on principles, goals and objectives it is a method of change in awareness through self healing, a process of transformation of consciousness as mindfulness in everyday life, an outcome of the transformative vision, and an objective of spiritual healing of identity as the self.

The method is based on the nursing theory of Rogers, the science that the universe is an energy field that transforms only, neuroscience that the brain changes structure and functioning as awareness changes, awareness that the unified field is an interconnected whole across time and space, the method of meditation on the levels as energy, a holistic model of health as our integration and a model of mental health nursing practice of the therapeutic use of self to recover identity and in doing so prevent crises occurring.

In the past the term "to remember" had religious significance of putting the parts of self together. Meditation is a neuroplastic exercise of putting the parts together as we remember the opening of the levels. We put the parts of self together as brain connects the parts. Brain connects the parts through belief in that occurring. To remember the transformative vision is to heal, to be made whole.

We are energy fields. That we and environment are interconnected energy fields is a scientific fact; otherwise we wouldn't exist. That meditation is a neuroplastic exercise of change in awareness is a fact. That we self heal as we become aware of the energy field is Roger's theory of nursing. The practice of mental health nursing is using self to assist change. Science, theory and practice are connected by Narrative Meditation as a method of self healing. The evidence of well being through empowerment is engagement in meditation and life as the forming of goals and objectives.

Change occurs through the method of how meditation is practiced. Mediation is learnt in stages. Meditation deepens as the energy field becomes known. Deeper levels of meditation are different levels of our individual, transpersonal, and spiritual healing. The levels are accessed as they have meaning as principles and purpose as goals that can be imagined as experience.

The goal at the apex is accessing the transformative vision. The experience is the transformation of consciousness as vision. The self is state of consciousness of vision. Vision as a state of consciousness is the energy of our whole selves. To be energy it has to be used. Mastery of Narrative Meditation is belief in identity as the self and a lifestyle decision. It is made in understanding of the possibilities of vision of mindfulness as a state of consciousness in everyday life, experience as healing, and spirituality as belief.

As experience mastery is a state of synchronicity of inner experience of healing of the levels, outer experience of transformation of the aspects and outer serendipitous events that assist us realise goals and objectives. Energy has to be used. Through the decision we are consciously using our energy field to change experience as an intention.

Through our stories of transformation of awareness, experience and belief another narrative has been evolving as there connection. The narrative that has been evolving is the remembering of the self. The transformative vision is awareness of the energy field. Movement into the energy field is through the decision of how to be. The aspect of belief is fully formed through belief in identity as the self.

The decision is to be of service in our circumstances. The decision is made in awareness of a crisis, possibilities as alternatives to that and how the crisis can be prevented. Individuals form culture and in turn awareness is collectively shaped by culture. The possibility is that individual self healing transforms collective awareness and experience through a renaissance. A renaissance transforms history.

Meditation is accessed through the transformative vision however mastery and spirituality may not be objectives. That does not mean that meditation is not accessible; that's not how it works. Meditation is accessible because it is learnt in stages. It is a process of development of principles, goals and objectives in awareness of possibilities. The outer journey is awareness of the transcendent possibilities of self healing of a renaissance of culture, prevention of mental illness and vision to achieve the transformation of awareness, experience, belief and identity.

There are two ways of approaching Narrative Meditation; as a method of change to self heal or as a method of transformation. The difference is awareness of possibilities. As personal art it is mental practice with the objective of self healing to achieve health and well being. To practice meditation with the possibility of transformation in this life and the next, it is spiritual practice. Whether we accept meditation as either personal art or spiritual practice to achieve our eventual final transformation is an individual decision. But beliefs are necessary for any level of healing and evolve as we ask questions.

As a guide this book is about meditation as a method of healing and transformation. The method is a process of transformation of consciousness as vision, an outcome of the transformative vision, and an objective of individual, transpersonal, and spiritual healing. Mastery is a lifestyle decision of how to be made in awareness of possibilities. The decision to identify as the self is the possibility of psyche's transformation.

My role as a guide is understanding Narrative Meditation as a guided meditation on principles to enable you to form your goals whatever they may be, because it's all about empowerment in awareness of change occurring. Understanding is not just getting your head around it; it is getting your head into it through change in awareness. Understanding the method and the transformative vision leads to you developing your own goals as a meditation. The hard part is the forming of goals and this we do in stages as we remember the transformative vision aided by a plan of our self as whole.

∞

This book is about psyche's transformation, what that is and how. A friend said to me understanding psyche is complex and people haven't got time to understand meditation, they just want to do it and anyway people already have access to guided meditation, groups and methods that have been around for decades so what is the purpose of this method? People would be more interested in an insider's stories about asylums so why not write about that?

I partially agreed. The interaction of body and emotions, thoughts and beliefs is complex to understand as the interaction of energy. Many people have had the unitary experience in meditation but have a different understanding of what it is to enable them to use it in everyday life. I believe that access to meditation and healing are connected with understanding of it... The self has been written about and meditation has been practiced for a very long time but I just couldn't enter the gate of the secret garden and I wanted to understand why; it wasn't my garden and I didn't know how to create it. Understanding is a process of change in awareness and experience.

As a guide this book is about reducing complexity by understanding the pyramid of life as a symbol of ourselves. Understanding our framework and how it is connected gives meditation on the transformative vision meaning as union and purpose of being made whole. This book is written for people who like me want understanding of what the garden is and from a nurse's perspective of how to create it. That's what you learn from participating in creating the asylum as a centre of rehabilitation.

Anyway the asylum has been written about already (Irving Goffman's, **Asylums**) but not how they changed. Medications changed but not the culture for over a hundred years despite the best intentions of many. The organisation changed as the culture changed. That changed as nurse's identity changed as expert mental health nurses. That's the real story of how change occurred.

I did focus groups to discuss what a model of mental health nursing practice was. They said that's what they already do even in forensic services; that's all I wanted to hear. It's always about facilitating recovery while being aware of all risks. Nurses no longer believed in identity as woogaroo screws, and anyway no one would want to hear negative stories about the asylum. No one would believe them and they are an indictment everyone would rather forget. Psychiatry taught that chronicity was inevitable. Society had accepted that recovery wasn't possible and that cultures are a given that can't be changed. The asylum was a mirror of the culture of society.

This book is written to people wherever they may be and of whatever beliefs you may have. It is written in the hope that if you like it, I can consider myself a writer. Vision develops as the artist learns how to connect with readers. A good writer in making connections inspires others.

Connections exist as awareness changes. Their existence changes experience. Stories are all about change in awareness, experience, and beliefs about that; that's what stories are. A good writer is a storyteller who in connecting them as a narrative gives our stories of change meaning and purpose.

The narrative of the remembering of the self unfolds as our stories are connected as psyche's journey of transformation of identity. Psyche can only be transformed through our own stories. I am a writer of a story of the remembering of the self. I become a creative writer when I inspire you to be the author of your story.

As a writer my books are stories of change in understanding. Through reflection on my roles, my practice as a nurse, changes in inner and outer circumstances I experienced inspiration. Inspiration is the connection of energy within self and between self and environment in the present moment. It's the creative experience; that's how I write and why I enjoy it. My understanding changed as I was remembering the transformative vision.

Psyche as what we are is a broad canvas on which we create. The broad canvas is our unconscious energy field on which we are creating our experience. What we create is a projection of what we are aware of psyche as being. Narrative Meditation is the art of change in psyche's awareness to create our experience. Experiencing the transformative vision of union is awareness that all things are connected.

In the present moment President Trump has created division with and between the EU; creating further polarisation in the US. At the same time a young soccer team is rescued due only to international cooperation which everyone is grateful for. The contrast of division and service, compassion, creativity, peace, love and connection with others winning the day and news headlines was stark. For the boys it confirmed their faith in Buddhism. For me it confirmed my belief in the power of principles to unite.

At the present moment critics of the President and the media have been sent parcel bombs. President Trump has blamed the media for causing national division. At home in Australia the elected Prime Minister has been sacked by conservatives of his own party which was described as a form of political madness. The madness is the self interest of ego gaining power through division. Because of his sacking an independent female was elected on a platform of addressing climate change and she holds the balance of power in parliament; the times they are a changing.

At present scientists are working out if time travel is possible by conceptualising the universe as a block of energy. They won't unless they conceptualise it as the unified field that is across all time and space. That's what change in understanding is all about. In Australia researchers are using goals and behavioural change as a neuroplastic intervention to change eating habits, using virtual reality as a neuroplastic intervention to treat addictions and treating dementia with music, dancing (some dance to remember some dance to forget) and virtual reality. The virtual reality displayed is connection with nature. In the present moment researchers at Griffith University are using virtual reality to assist heal spinal injuries. I hope they work as interventions but they are not neuroplastic exercises of change in awareness, experience, and belief. I believe meditation should also be used as part of a recovery program.

In the present there are calls by prominent psychiatrists for a Royal Commission to fix cracks in the mental health system caused by deinstitutionalisation. It is recognised in Australia there is a mental health crisis among youth. Systems can be improved but the problem can only be fixed through funding education programs to prevent mental health crises occurring. In the present moment Hurricane Michael has devastated 4 states in the USA and Al Gore said if we don't address the UN report on climate change it could be the end of civilisation. 60% of the media in Australia made no mention of the report. Elon Musk is conducting an outer space program to colonise Mars in case the Earth becomes uninhabitable. I believe it will be unless we conquer inner space first.

At present the Duke and Duchess of Sussex, Prince Harry and Meghan are sponsoring the **Invictus Games,** symbolised by the logo, **I Am.** What is recovered for disabled veterans through their goals and extraordinary achievements is identity. They are also promoting recovery from mental illness through lifestyle change. Both groups face the same issue of recovery of identity through vision of a meaningful life. Principles of the royals are shining through which most Australians like. The Queen has announced a Commonwealth Canopy of protected forests across 53 nations which environmentally aware people also like. The rebranding of the royal family as serving society and the planet has broad appeal. What

am I saying? I believe in an Ausralian republic. Australians collectively
don't yet have an identity; we are still in adolescence as an independent
nation because the Queen still has the power to dismiss the government.
Identity matters at an individual, and collective level.

At present blended honey like identity as ego is fake and similarly no
one was aware of that occurring. At the same time it is the best honey flow
in years and real honey like vision is medicinal. I

In the present moment, collectively psyche is split in our culture. The
split was said to be between the reasoning of technique and creativity; it's
deeper than that. Psyche is split between identity as ego and the self. We
cling to ego because we think the alternative is a void of nothingness when
it isn't; the contrary is true. The void is a state of alienation in awareness
of identity as ego. The split is resolved through psyche's transformation.
Ego exists as continuity of materialism. The self exists as continuity
of transformation. Our story changes as we do and that's the journey.
The quest is to remember the self to create who we are. The quest is to
remember the self.

∞

As a guide I have been writing about the sublime. Mastery is a lifestyle
decision in circumstances which usually don't appear all that ethereal.
Goals and objectives form our identity of what we are, who we are, and
believe ourselves to be. As a guide I am a writer. As a guide and a writer
I am a person. The goal of assisting others self heal, becoming a creative
writer and personal goals were connected.

While creating my books I was thinking about my roles in the past
as a nurse, in the present as a guide, and my role as a writer of a possible
future; they were interacting if you haven't noticed. Awareness of the past
and vision for the future creates who we are. Integrated they are who I am
as a person.

My objective is to maximise my and others potential for health, well
being and happiness through being of service as a guide, a writer and as
a person. A goal had always been to serve the land; a promise I made to
an aboriginal elder as traditional owners of the country where I live. In
serving the land we heal through awareness of connection with it. I came
to understand self as I did; that's what aboriginal spirituality of awareness
of connection is and what female healing country does.

63

Meditation has been a tool that adjusts as understanding, experience and circumstances change. In awareness of how to remember the transformative vision and the possibility of the strength in reach of vision to change inner and outer circumstances I changed my meditation. It is tribal Gubbi Gubbi land but also my home and retreat. I teach meditation through writing and to people individually but now have an expanded vision. I changed my goal of use of the land to establishing a meditation school. In awareness of this goal I am the self my objective.

∞

I had inspiring thoughts over many years of creating a retreat but that hasn't transpired because of reasoning that it was beyond my means but may as the parts come together through vision of it as a school. As in meditation goals and objectives are achieved in stages. It is a school when people come to learn Narrative Meditation to become transformative therapists.

The school would be based on principles of the levels, using science, art, and spirituality to achieve creative goals. Experts would be invited to practice awareness of the levels to assist understanding. Partnership would be invited with community groups and traditional owners to share their culture and knowledge. The objective of the school is developing awareness through meditation. I may have to settle for another goal of beekeeping but on another level they are similar.

I had become aware of a bee crisis that was worldwide but had no knowledge or skills so have been learning different methods. Beekeeping and teaching meditation are similar as assisting change and transformation. For beekeepers assisting the change of nectar into honey enables a transformation of larvae to bees. What makes this possible is the framework of the hive is an integrated whole connected with its environment. Teaching assists change of the nectar of consciousness into the honey of vision to enable a transformation of identity. What makes this possible is the framework of the self is an integrated whole in awareness of the transformative vision of connection with environment.

The bee crisis is an environmental crisis. The crisis of consciousness is a cultural crisis. Both teaching and beekeeping have similar purpose of improving the whole environment in which we live to prevent crises

———

occurring. They are both about the possibility of improving circumstances for others.

Bees have roles but collectively they are a hive that pollinates the environment. The possibility is that collectively transformative visionaries pollinate a cultural renaissance. It occurs through the splitting of hives of sharing the honey between many as we use what we have, and share what we get in awareness of possibilities. The trick is knowing when the bees are about to swarm; I didn't but there's always a new spring.

As a novice beekeeper, I was learning how to go inside the hive. As keepers of our energy field, we learn how to go inside using our strength in reach of vision to change inner and outer circumstances. Whether to establish a retreat or an apiary is all about making connections and believing in possibilities that are not exclusive.

Why is the quest of remembering identity important? Vision of goals of our whole selves forms it and energy has to be used. The levels are opened by the self using vision. At the 8th level of awareness of the transformative vision, identity connects inner and outer circumstances. I changed my meditation to include all goals that were connected with principles, objectives and inspired me in the present moment, could be imagined as experience. For me it goes like this;

At the red level of body and service, I serve my body through health goals of being fit, healthy, and pain free; I serve nature through creating Gaia as a beautiful place through revegetation and beekeeping; I serve others through working as a successful writer. My body is relaxed.

At the orange level of emotions and compassion, in gratitude for health and lifestyle I have empathy with others suffering physically, emotionally, mentally and spiritually through alienation and act compassionately by giving support and teaching meditation to assist self healing. My emotions are calm.

At the yellow level of thought and creativity, I use my inspiration to achieve creative goals of the personal arts, and creating a meditation school. I stilled my thoughts to allow the energy of all inspirational goals of health, writing, teaching and creating in.

At the green level of belief and peace, in relaxation, calmness of emotions and stillness of thought, I meditated on belief in the peace of inner silence as healing.

At the blue level of love and presence, love is expressing as unconditional service, compassion, creativity and peace. Blue is for presence.

At the indigo level of connection and beauty, I connect with my environment through presence. Indigo is for the beauty of connection with home, pets, nature, the elements, the mountains and valleys, my community and society.

At the violet level of spirit and others, spirit is energy between us, between me my family, friends, the sick, parents and teachers that inspires a vision of renaissance. I meditate on belief in spirit as love.

The eighth level has meaning as union with the energy field and purpose as the transformation of identity. We have been using the symbol of the pyramid to assist transformation. The self is state of consciousness of vision of goals of the levels. There merging at the 8th level forms identity. What now is the symbol of the self?

The pyramid of life transforms as the star within. The star as light merges with the unified field where there is no past, present or future as time or space as objects. Where there is no time or objects is the transformative vision of the unified field. That's what union with the field is and how the state of meditation is accessed. In meditation on this symbol we are the self; a state of consciousness of vision of the transcendence of time and space.

Imagine the white apex
White is for identity and union
The colours merge transforming the pyramid as the star within
Light of the star fills the universe Flowing into the past before time began
Into the future and Afterlife
Meditate on the transformative vision
The unified field

∞

What this book is about is answered when we ask what has changed? We are aware that consciousness is energy already through experiences in everyday life of connection of consciousness and experience. We rationalise, deny or forget them because they don't fit with collective beliefs and our identity as ego. In moments of connection we know this is true but vision must be of use before we accept the self as what and who we are. The self is remembered to heal.

This book is about a method of meditation to remember identity. Spiritual healing is identity as the self. The self is what we are as an energy field, who we are as experience, and believe ourselves to be; the inner and outer are connected. The self is state of consciousness of vision, of mindfulness of goals and objectives of our whole selves. This book is about empowerment to achieve them using meditation as mental or spiritual practice. The inner journey is to the transformative vision of wholeness and unity, awareness of connection of self and self with environment. The outer journey is to awareness of the possibilities of vision. What now is the possibility of transformation of identity as the self?

The ultimate possibility of identity as the self, and the most hopeful, is living from the inside. The transformative vision is spiritual healing. Spiritual healing is a state of empowerment in awareness of ourselves as whole in the present moment. The present moment is where past and future meet; always has been, always will be and always is the eternal now. The eternal now is accessed through the transformative vision of the unified field and as vision in everyday life. Living in the present moment is living from the inside. Mastery of meditation is belief in identity as the self and a way of being of living from the inside. What is changing is living from the inside; the eighth possibility of vision.

The hopeful part is change in our experience to maximise our potential. The energy of the self only exists in the present moment where the past and future meet. Where past and future meet is the unified field. How we access that is through meditation and in mindfulness of goals and objectives, we are the self; the connection of the inner and the outer. The possibility is we access the energy of the self by living from the inside; the star is released by the transformative vision.

The original question was how do we use vision in everyday life? That question and the question of what the self is are the same. The self is state of consciousness of vision. Vision as mindfulness of goals and objectives in the present moment is living from the inside. Living from the inside changes the experience of daily living. This is the answer to the question and what our quest of remembering the self is all about.

∞

As a nurse the objective was using self to inspire vision of a meaningful life. That occurred through a plan to assist the forming of goals as a method of change and transformation. Awareness of what the self is changed through experience and meditation.

———

As a guide the first objective of this book is understanding the self. Narrative Meditation as a method is a process, an outcome and objectives that are transforming awareness, experience and belief to achieve possibilities. The first objective of this book is understanding what the self is as the energy of vision, how we access it through meditation and use it as mindfulness of goals and objectives. Understanding is a change in awareness. The first objective is a change in awareness.

My understanding of the self took a long time. It took a long time as awareness, and experience changed, and belief that identity is their connection developed. Through understanding what the self is your journey has started and has a destination.

The second objective of this book is access to the state of meditation and healing. The first and second objectives are connected. The state of meditation is accessed through the transformative vision of there being no time or objects. Understanding what the self is, and how we access and use it gives the transformative vision meaning as the state of meditation and purpose as healing. The second objective is a change in experience.

As a nurse the objective of the therapeutic use of self was to assist change through a vision of well being. This vision inspired engagement of patients in the forming of goals and objectives. As a guide it is to assist understanding what the self and the transformative vision is so the self can be remembered. As a writer my objective is to be inspirational.

If this book inspires you to experience the transformative vision, what is inspirational is remembering your own vision. Through understanding the transformative vision the state of meditation is accessed. What has changed is vision is remembered. What changes is experience as healing.

Healing occurs as a neuroplastic intervention as we remember the experience of the transformative vision. As we are empowered through change we are inspired to form goals enabling healing of the levels, access to deeper levels of meditation, and transformation of the aspects to maximise our potential. Through the decision what changes is identity as the self.

∞

Someone raised a question about imagining the transformative vision and through imagining what is in fact real we experience the unified field. Then I said the levels are opened by the self. He asked; then it wasn't imagined, wasn't it in fact real as the energy of consciousness? I replied yes, they are both correct. In the beginning we use the imagination. As identity changes we remember that it is the energy of the self, vision that is opening the levels.

At the 8ᵗʰ level the energy of the self connects with our whole environment. That's what the unified field is. That's what the transformation of belief in identity does. He then said we experience the transformative vision in meditation but the unified field is limitless consisting of enormous events, black holes, billions of stars whose light does not reach us and if it did they may be long dead, and extraordinary beauty so how can we really be aware of it, let alone experience it?

The energy field is a unified whole across time and space. Awareness of it as these events locates you as a state of consciousness in time. Awareness of it as a unified field is a different state of consciousness of the archetypal image of wholeness and unity; the transformative vision. The transformative vision of union is awareness that all things are connected. The unified field is localised as a very small place of connections occurring in the present moment. That's what the unified field is and what the transformative vision does. As in the inner is the outer is a state of consciousness of vision.

Someone else asked me recently do I now remember past lives? We have all been here before but I don't remember identity in past lives. Objectives are echoes from past lives to remember the self in this life. Past lives are part of the journey of finding our way home. Another said to me access to meditation through the transformative vision could be beneficial for the spiritual needs of people in palliative care. This raised the possibility there are many applications of the remembering of the self; the transformative vision heals. Healing occurs on different levels depending on objectives of individual, transpersonal and spiritual healing.

These comments also raised the possibility there are more questions for me as a guide, and hopefully as a writer. As a person life goes on in mindfulness as a pleasing aesthetic, spiritual and practical way of being. For me, living from the inside is awareness of connection.

My happiness is when visitors bring delightful food, wine, music, and insights from connecting with the landscape, nature, and me as a person. I connect with others through talking about their goals and objectives to achieve their vision of well being. It's a learnt way of how to be and I don't want to be any other way. I am the self, my objective in awareness of connection with others. The other is the self in awareness that I am the self. A healer inspires remembering of the self, that's what a transformative therapist does; use self to inspire goals and objectives and use them as a meditation on remembering of the self. Like any expert nurse knows the job isn't done till what is happening is documented. For people on a quest of transformation the documentation is a journal of inspiration and change using a narrative approach to meditation.

Living from the inside feels right to me, like finally coming home to where I belong. As a novice beekeeper, going to harvest honey for the first time, living from the inside is useful. Being centred in mindfulness is my way of going inside the hive and that now doesn't involve a decision, it's simply a learnt way of being, of living from the inside.

∞

Psyche's transformation is identity as the self. The self can only be remembered through our own stories. Stories have a beginning, a middle, and an end. This story began with awareness of the transformative vision. Our life story unfolds as the energy of vision connects awareness, experience, and belief. The narrative that is unfolding is the transformation of identity. Belief in identity as a state of quantum consciousness of vision ends this story of remembering the self.

24th October, 2018